DIABETIC DIET COOKBOOK FOR BEGINNERS AND NEWLY DIAGNOSED

30-Day Delicious Snacks, Tasty Recipes, and Easy Meal Plans, Featuring Vegetarian Pasta Options

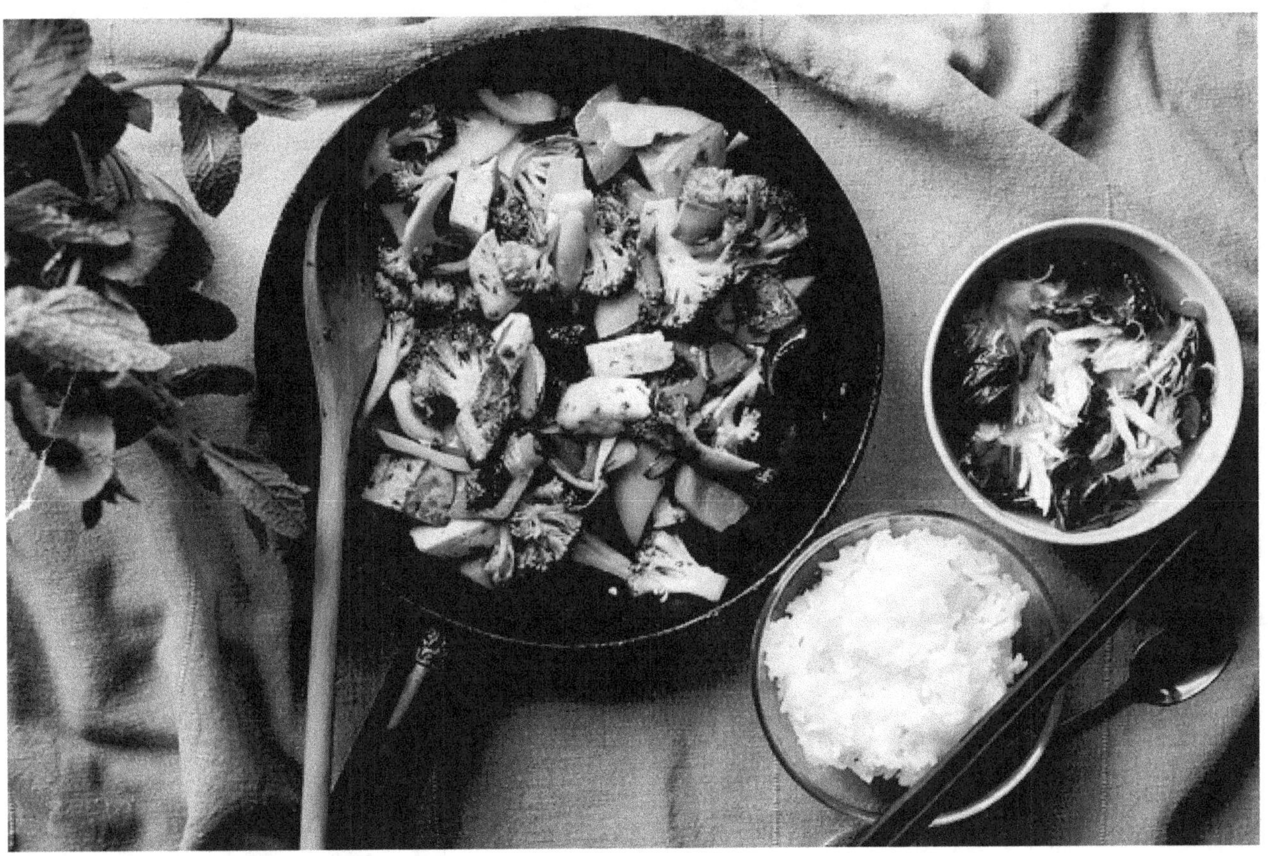

Anissa T.Wasinger

OTHER BOOKS BY ANISSA T.WASINGER

AIR FRYER COOKBOOK FOR BEGINNERS SUPER DELICIOUS PLANT-POWERED COOKBOOK FOR BUSY FAMILIES WITH IMAGES

KINDLY SCAN THE QR CODE TO GIVE YOUR HONEST REVIEW.

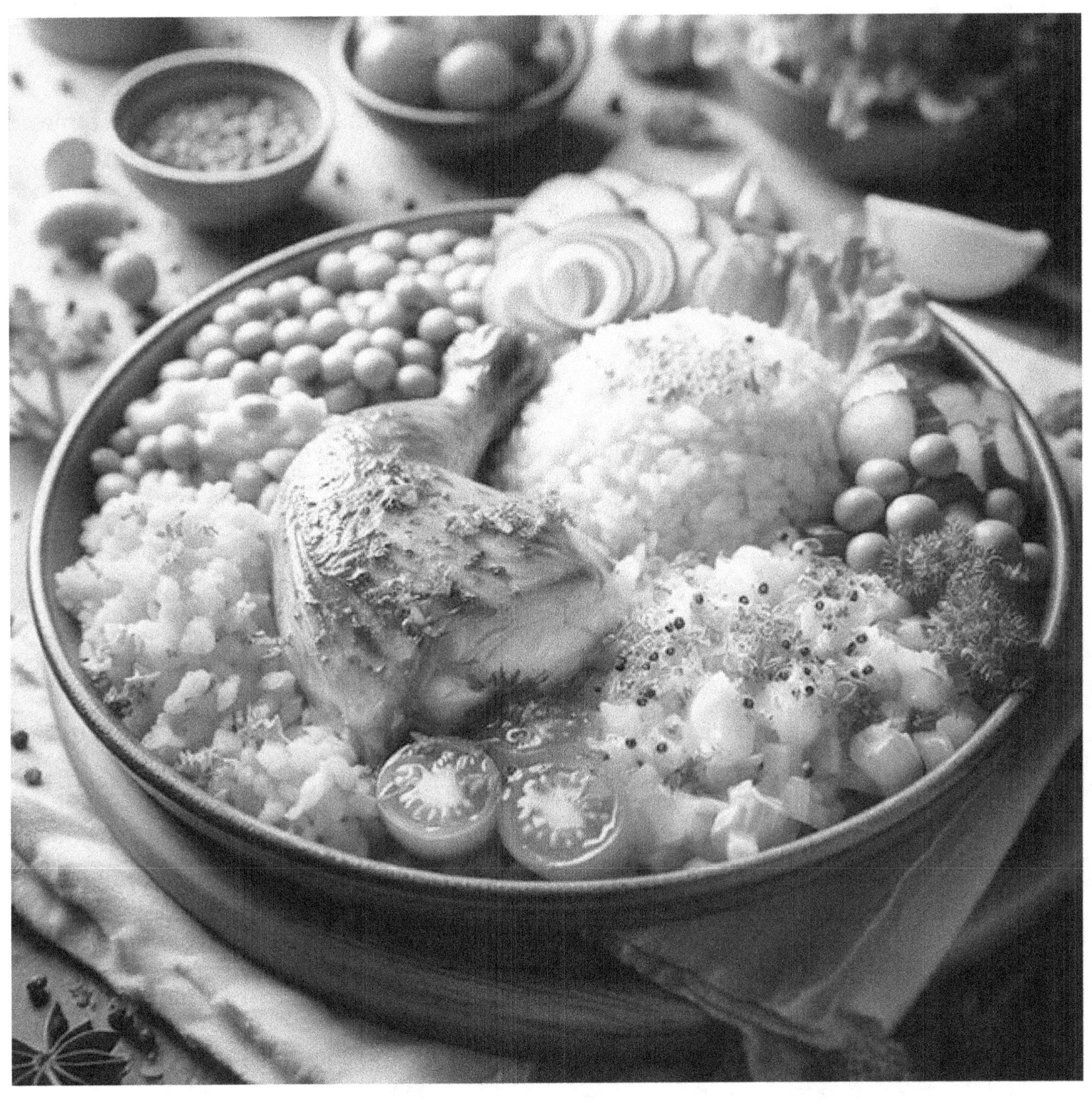

Greetings and welcome to the path of health transformation and gastronomic empowerment! This cookbook is a veritable gold mine of information, recipes, and tips carefully crafted to help you navigate the complex world of diabetes diet. As a practicing physician and nutritionist, I have personally experienced the confusing maze that a diabetes diagnosis may bring. However, I've also witnessed the incredible resiliency and growth potential that surface with the correct knowledge and resources.

Together, let's set out on this journey equipped with recipes, understanding, feeling, and a hint of confusion because the world of diabetes can be very confusing.

What is diabetes exactly? It's a complicated combination of elements that can change connections with food and shape lives, making it more than just a medical illness. Fundamentally, diabetes is a metabolic disease marked by high blood sugar levels, which are either the consequence of inadequate insulin synthesis or inefficient insulin use by the body. But it's a process that forces us to reconsider how we approach nutrition and lifestyle—it's more than just numbers on a glucose meter.

We'll cover all the different kinds of diabetes in these pages, from the well-known Type 1 and Type 2 to the less common varieties like MODY (Maturity-Onset Diabetes of the Young) and the frequently misdiagnosed gestational diabetes. We'll address them with compassion and transparency. Every kind has unique considerations and difficulties.

The main source of our life, food may also be a cause of uncertainty and irritation for those who are managing their diabetes. Do not be alarmed; this is not only a list of dos and don'ts; rather, it is a guide to preparing tasty and healthful meals. We'll look at the diverse range of foods that can help you on your path to optimum health and also identify some that could backfire.

However, this cookbook is a manifesto for prevention and control rather than merely a compilation of recipes. We'll dive into the habits and techniques that can help you take control of your health, such as the value of consistent exercise and mindful eating. Together, we'll discover the keys to living well with diabetes rather than merely managing it.

So be ready, reader, for a culinary journey unlike any other. Let us welcome the voyage with reason, feeling, and, perhaps, a little confusion. Because everything in these pages has the potential to change not just the way you eat but the way you think about health and wellbeing in general. Welcome to the Diabetic Diet Cookbook for Newly Diagnosed and Beginners, where empowerment is king and delicious meets nutritious. Together, let's create a culinary storm for our well-being, joy, and longevity!

What is the sound of that?

What is diabetes?

Diabetes is a complex metabolic illness that affects people on a physical, emotional, and social level. Diabetes is characterized by chronically increased blood sugar levels, which are caused by either insufficient insulin synthesis by the pancreas or defective insulin action. This metabolic imbalance is the foundation of a complex interaction of physiological and behavioral factors that together create the diabetes experience.

Recognizing the many kinds of diabetes is critical to comprehending it. Type 1 diabetes, which is often diagnosed in childhood or adolescence, is caused by autoimmune loss of insulin-producing beta cells in the pancreas, necessitating lifelong insulin therapy. Type 2 diabetes, which is more common in adults but is increasingly affecting younger people, is distinguished by insulin resistance, in which cells fail to respond effectively to insulin signals, as well as growing beta cell failure. Gestational diabetes, which develops during pregnancy, presents special challenges for both the mother and the child, while other kinds, such as MODY (Maturity-Onset Diabetes of the Young), highlight the genetic variety of the disorder.

Diabetes affects all aspects of daily living, including food, exercise, and healthcare. It necessitates close monitoring of blood glucose levels, precise medication management, and adherence to dietary and lifestyle changes. Diabetes, however, is distinguished not just by its obstacles, but also by the human spirit's perseverance and flexibility.

Diabetes is a transforming experience, not just a diagnosis. It's an invitation to embrace empowerment, question assumptions, and rethink ideas about health and well-being. It serves as a reminder that our bodies are more than just channels for disease; they also contain potential and resiliency. Individuals with diabetes can manage this road with courage and confidence by receiving knowledge, support, and compassionate care that turns adversity into opportunity and uncertainty into empowerment.

Types of Diabetes

Type One Diabetes:

Type 1 diabetes, often known as juvenile diabetes, is an autoimmune disorder in which the body's immune system erroneously assaults and destroys insulin-producing beta cells in the pancreas. This autoimmune attack causes a severe reduction or complete halt of insulin production, culminating in total insulin insufficiency. Individuals with Type 1 diabetes rely on exogenous insulin injections or insulin pumps to control their blood sugar levels. This type of diabetes often appears in childhood or adolescence, but it can occur at any age. While the specific origin of Type 1 diabetes is unknown, genetic predisposition and environmental factors are thought to play important roles.

Type 2 diabetes:

Type 2 diabetes, the most common type of diabetes globally, is defined by insulin resistance - a disease in which cells fail to respond effectively to insulin signals - combined with increasing beta cell malfunction, which leads to decreased insulin output over time. Unlike Type 1 diabetes, which has an autoimmune component, Type 2 diabetes is caused mostly by a genetic predisposition, lifestyle factors (such as sedentary behavior and bad eating habits), and obesity. While Type 2 diabetes is more common in adults, it is being diagnosed in younger people as obesity and sedentary lifestyles become more prevalent. Type 2 diabetes is normally managed with lifestyle changes, oral medicines, and, in some circumstances, insulin therapy.

Gestational Diabetes:

Gestational diabetes mellitus (GDM) is characterized by high blood sugar levels that appear or are first detected during pregnancy. While the precise mechanisms driving gestational diabetes remain unknown, hormonal changes during pregnancy, together with preexisting insulin resistance, contribute to its development. GDM endangers both the mother and the growing fetus, including macrosomia (high birth weight), birth difficulties, and a higher chance of developing Type 2 diabetes later in life for both mother and child. Dietary adjustments, blood glucose monitoring, and, in rare circumstances, insulin therapy are used to manage the condition.

Maturity-Onset Diabetes in the Young (MODY):

Maturity-Onset Diabetes of the Young (MODY) is a subset of monogenic diabetes defined by autosomal dominant heredity and frequently diagnosed before the age of 25. MODY is caused by mutations in certain genes that control beta cell activity and insulin release, resulting in variable degrees of poor glucose regulation. MODY, unlike Type 1 and Type 2 diabetes, is rare and frequently misdiagnosed due to its unusual presentation and genetic variability. MODY management entails genetic testing to ensure an accurate diagnosis and appropriate therapy options.

Other types of diabetes:

In addition to the aforementioned types, there are other less common forms of diabetes, such as secondary diabetes caused by other medical conditions (such as pancreatitis or cystic fibrosis), drug-induced diabetes (caused by certain medications), and monogenic diabetes that differs from MODY.

Each kind of diabetes poses unique problems and considerations, emphasizing the significance of personalized management strategies adapted to individual requirements and circumstances. Understanding the differences between each kind is critical for developing successful treatment and prevention methods, as well as delivering comprehensive care to people with diabetes.

<u>10 comprehensive ways to prevent and control diabetes</u>

1. Maintain a healthy weight:

Achieving and maintaining a healthy weight through a balanced diet and regular physical activity is critical for preventing and controlling diabetes. Excess body weight, particularly abdominal fat, leads to insulin resistance and an increased risk of developing Type 2 diabetes.

2. Maintain a Balanced Diet:

Consume fruits, vegetables, whole grains, lean proteins, and healthy fats, while minimizing refined carbohydrates, sugary drinks, and processed meals. Adopting a Mediterranean-style diet, often known as the DASH diet (Dietary Approaches to Stop Hypertension), has shown promise in terms of lowering the risk of diabetes and increasing blood sugar control.

3. Track Carbohydrate Intake:

Carbohydrates have the greatest impact on blood sugar levels, therefore it's critical to monitor carbohydrate intake and choose complex carbohydrates with a low glycemic index to help keep blood sugar stable. Fiber-rich diets can also aid reduce glucose absorption and improve blood sugar regulation.

4. Regular physical activity

Improves insulin sensitivity, decreases blood sugar levels, and promotes healthy weight management. Aim for at least 150 minutes of moderate-intensity aerobic activity or 75 minutes of vigorous-intensity activity per week, with muscle-strengthening activities on two or more days.

5. Monitor blood sugar levels:

Regular blood sugar monitoring provides vital insights into glycemic control and helps identify trends and patterns that may necessitate changes to treatment approaches. Collaborate with your healthcare team to define target blood sugar ranges and create a monitoring routine that is tailored to your specific needs.

6. Manage stress levels:

Chronic stress can raise blood sugar levels and lead to insulin resistance, so stress management is an important aspect of diabetes prevention and control. Use relaxation techniques like deep breathing, meditation, yoga, or hobbies to reduce stress and increase general well-being.

7. Get quality sleep:

Inadequate or interrupted sleep can affect hormone levels, particularly insulin, and impair glucose metabolism. Prioritize obtaining enough, high-quality sleep every night, aiming for 7-9 hours for most adults.

8. Limit alcohol intake:

Excessive alcohol intake can disturb blood sugar levels and interfere with medication effectiveness. It's crucial to consume alcohol in moderation or abstain entirely, especially if you have diabetes or are at risk of acquiring it.

9. Quit smoking:

To reduce the risk of Type 2 diabetes and its consequences, including cardiovascular disease. Seek help and resources for quitting smoking and improving your general health.

10. Regular medical check-ups,

Screening for diabetes risk factors and complications, is crucial for early detection, intervention, and treatment of the condition. Stay proactive in controlling your health by making regular appointments with your healthcare team and actively participating in your treatment plan.

These comprehensive strategies include lifestyle changes, food choices, and proactive healthcare procedures to help individuals prevent and control diabetes.

Dietary Requirements

1. Carbohydrate Management:

Carbohydrates have the greatest impact on blood sugar levels, hence, it is critical to monitor and control carbohydrate intake. Choose complex carbs with a low glycemic index, such as whole grains, legumes, fruits, and vegetables, which are digested more slowly and result in gradual blood sugar increases. Limit your intake of refined carbs, sugary beverages, and processed foods, as these might cause your blood sugar to rise.

2. Portion Control:

Avoid overeating, which can lead to weight gain and high blood sugar levels. Use measuring cups, food scales, or visual cues to determine the right portion sizes for different food groups. Aim for balanced meals that include a variety of nutrient-dense foods in suitable serving sizes.

3. Balanced Diet:

Eat nutrient-dense foods from all dietary groups, such as fruits, vegetables, whole grains, lean meats, and healthy fats. To keep your blood sugar constant and avoid spikes and crashes, spread out your calorie consumption throughout the day.

4. Fiber Intake:

Consume more fiber to help with blood sugar regulation, satiety, and digestive health. Select fiber-rich foods such as fruits, vegetables, whole grains, legumes, nuts, and seeds. Aim for 25-30 grams of fiber each day, from both soluble and insoluble sources.

5. Healthy fats:

Include healthy fats in your diet, such as monounsaturated and polyunsaturated fats, to promote heart health and insulin sensitivity. Avocados, almonds, seeds, olive oil, fatty salmon, and flaxseed are all good sources of healthy fats. Limit saturated and trans fats, which are present in fried foods, processed snacks, and fatty meats, and can raise the risk of heart disease.

6. Protein Sources:

Incorporate lean protein sources into your meals to boost satiety, improve muscular health, and balance blood sugar levels. Choose lean meats, chicken, fish, tofu, tempeh, lentils, and low-fat dairy products. Protein should be consumed equally throughout the day to maximize muscle protein synthesis and blood sugar regulation.

7. Stay hydrated

By drinking plenty of water throughout the day. Water regulates blood sugar levels, promotes kidney function, and assists digestion. Limit your intake of sugary beverages, caffeinated beverages, and alcohol, which can lead to dehydration and alter blood sugar management.

8. Sodium Reduction:

Limit salt intake to improve heart health and lower the risk of high blood pressure and cardiovascular problems. When available, choose low-sodium or sodium-free products, and instead of salt, add flavor using herbs, spices, citrus juices, and vinegar. Aim to take no more than 2,300 milligrams of salt per day, and considerably less if you have hypertension or other risk factors.

9. Meal Time and Frequency:

To assist in stabilizing blood sugar levels and avoiding excessive fluctuations, stick to a steady meal plan and distribute your calories equally throughout the day. To maintain stable energy levels and glycemic management, eat every 3-4 hours and incorporate a variety of carbohydrates, protein, and fat at each meal and snack.

To manage diabetes effectively, consult with a qualified dietitian or healthcare professional to create a personalized dietary plan based on your unique needs, tastes, and lifestyle. Monitor blood sugar levels regularly and change your diet as needed to maintain optimal glycemic management and general well-being.

These dietary needs serve as a foundation for optimal diabetes management while also improving general health and well-being. By implementing these ideas into your dietary habits, you can improve blood sugar control, avoid difficulties, and live a healthier life.

Foods To Eat As a Diabetic Patient

1. Non-starchy vegetables:

Non-starchy veggies have little carbohydrates and calories but are high in important minerals, fiber, and antioxidants. Examples include leafy greens (spinach, kale, lettuce), cruciferous vegetables (broccoli, cauliflower, Brussels sprouts), peppers, cucumbers, zucchini, and tomatoes. Incorporating non-starchy veggies into meals increases volume, flavor, and nutrition without dramatically affecting blood sugar.

2. Whole Grains:

Whole grains are a great source of complex carbohydrates, fiber, vitamins, and minerals. They digest more slowly than refined carbohydrates, which helps to keep blood sugar levels stable. Choose whole grains such as quinoa, brown rice, barley, bulgur, oats, whole wheat, and buckwheat. These grains provide long-lasting energy, increase satiety, and improve digestive health.

3. Lean Proteins:

Lean protein sources help develop and repair tissues, promote muscle health, and stabilize blood sugar levels. Choose lean cuts of meat, chicken without skin, fish, seafood, tofu, tempeh, low-fat dairy products, eggs, and legumes. Including lean proteins in meals and snacks promotes fullness and avoids overeating.

4. Fatty Fish:

Fatty fish including salmon, mackerel, sardines, trout, and herring provide omega-3 fatty acids that promote heart health and reduce inflammation. Consuming fatty fish daily may help minimize the risk of cardiovascular disease, which is prevalent among diabetics. Aim to eat fatty fish at least twice a week.

5. Berries:

Strawberries, blueberries, raspberries, and blackberries are low in calories and carbs, but high in vitamins, minerals, fiber, and antioxidants. Berries have a low glycemic index, therefore they have little effect on blood sugar levels. Berries are a wholesome and delicious complement to breakfast, snacks, and desserts.

6. Nuts and Seeds:

Nuts and seeds are nutrient-dense foods that contain healthful fats, protein, fiber, vitamins, and minerals. They give long-lasting energy, increase satiety, and improve heart health. Unsalted nuts and seeds include almonds, walnuts, pistachios, peanuts, chia seeds, flaxseeds, and pumpkin seeds. Enjoy them as a snack, sprinkle them on salads or yogurt, or include them in recipes.

7. Legumes:

Beans, lentils, chickpeas, and peas are rich in plant-based protein, fiber, vitamins, and minerals. They have a low glycemic index and can help regulate blood sugar levels, induce satiety, and improve digestive health. Add beans to soups, salads, stews, casseroles, and grain bowls for a healthful and satisfying dinner.

8. Greek Yogurt

Greek yogurt is a protein-rich dairy food that contains critical elements like calcium, potassium, and vitamin D. It has a lower carbohydrate and greater protein content than conventional yogurt, making it a good choice for people with diabetes. To add flavor and texture, choose plain, unsweetened Greek yogurt and top it with fresh fruit, nuts, or seeds of your choice.

9. Avocado:

Avocado is a nutrient-dense fruit that contains heart-healthy monounsaturated fats, fiber, vitamins, and minerals. It has a low glycemic index and can aid with satiety and blood sugar control when added to meals and snacks. Avocado is deliciously sliced on toast, mixed into salads, blended into smoothies, or used as a spread instead of butter or mayonnaise.

10. Cinnamon:

A delicious spice with antioxidant and anti-inflammatory qualities, can enhance insulin sensitivity and reduce blood sugar levels. Sprinkle cinnamon over oatmeal, yogurt, smoothies, or baked goods for a tasty and nutritional boost.

These meals are nutrient-dense, low in carbohydrates, and have little effect on blood sugar levels, making them good choices for those with diabetes. Incorporating these foods into your diet will help you maintain good health, enhance glycemic control, and lower your risk of diabetic complications.

Foods To Avoid As a Diabetic Patient

1. Sugar-filled Drinks:

Due to their high sugar content, sugary drinks including soda, fruit juices, energy drinks, and sweetened teas can quickly raise blood sugar levels. They have little to no nutritional value and only give empty calories. Instead, go for water, unsweetened tea, or sparkling water with lime or lemon flavoring.

2. Refined Grains:

During processing, fiber and nutrients from refined grains, such as white bread, white rice, pasta, and pastries, are removed, which causes a sharp spike in blood sugar levels. Instead, choose whole grains, which have a slower effect on blood sugar and offer more fiber, vitamins, and minerals.

3. Snacks that have been processed and packaged:

Snacking options including chips, cookies, crackers, and snack bars are processed and packaged foods that are frequently heavy in added sugars, bad fats, and refined carbohydrates. They are linked to increased blood sugar, insulin resistance, and weight gain. Choose unprocessed, entire snacks like homemade trail mix, hummus-topped veggies, fresh fruit, and nuts.

4. Sweet Treats:

Because of their high sugar and refined carbohydrate content, sugary sweets including cakes, cookies, pies, ice cream, and candy can have a disastrous effect on blood sugar regulation. They lead to weight gain and insulin resistance, and they offer empty calories. Desserts are fine in moderation but choose healthier options like dark chocolate, fruit-based desserts, or homemade confections sweetened with stevia or monk fruit.

5. Fried Foods:

Fried foods include onion rings, french fries, fried chicken, and fried snacks that are heavy in calories, salt, and bad fats. They may increase the risk of cardiovascular disease, weight gain, and insulin resistance. Use heart-healthy cooking techniques like baking, grilling, steaming, or sautéing while using oils like avocado or olive oil.

6. Sugar-Rich Cereals for Breakfast:

Sweet breakfast cereals with added sugars and refined grains that are labeled as "kid-friendly" or "low-fat" frequently have little nutritional value and quickly raise blood sugar levels. To help regulate blood sugar levels, choose high-fiber, whole-grain cereals with little added sugar and serve them with meals strong in protein, such as almonds or Greek yogurt.

7. Yogurts with added sugar:

Yogurts that have been sweetened or flavored with fruit preserves, syrups, or additional sugars can have high sugar content and raise blood sugar levels. Choose low-fat or plain Greek yogurt without added sugar, and then, in moderation, top with your flavorings like nuts, seeds, or fresh fruit, as well as a drizzle of honey or maple syrup.

8. Processed meats :

Bacon, sausage, hot dogs, deli meats, canned meats, and other processed meats are heavy in sodium, harmful fats, and preservatives. They have been connected to higher risks of diabetes, cancer, and cardiovascular disease. For healthier protein sources, choose lean, unprocessed meats like skinless chicken, fish, tofu, or lentils.

9. Sugary Sauces & Condiments:

Sugary sauces and condiments, like sweet chili sauce, teriyaki sauce, barbecue sauce, and ketchup, can add empty calories and hidden sugars to food. Use sugar-free or low-sugar substitutes sparingly, or prepare your dressings and sauces with stevia or monk fruit, which are natural sweeteners.

10. Foods High in Sodium:

Foods heavy in sodium, like processed meats, canned soups, fast food, frozen dinners, and salty snacks, can raise blood pressure and the risk of cardiovascular disease, particularly in those with diabetes who are already at a higher risk. When possible, use low- or no-sodium options; in place of salt, season your food with herbs, spices, citrus juices, and vinegar.

By avoiding certain items, people can better control their blood sugar levels, enhance their general health, and lower their chance of developing diabetes-related problems. Rather, concentrate on nutrient-dense, whole foods that assist in steady blood sugar regulation and enhance general health.

CHAPTER 1

BREAKFAST RECIPES

1. Omelet of vegetables:

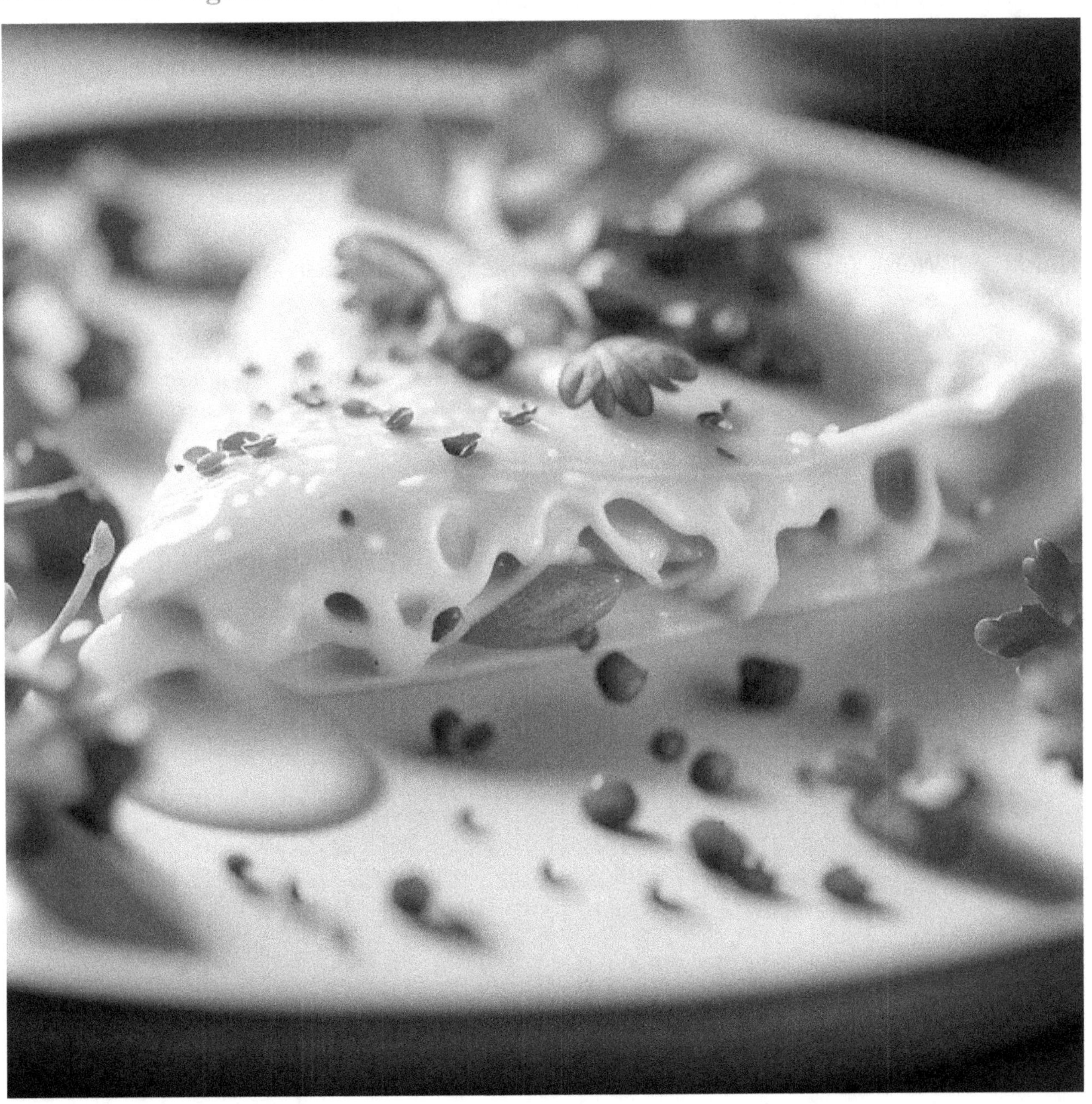

Components:
- Two eggs
- 1/4 cup of bell peppers, chopped
- 1/4 cup finely chopped onions
- 1/4 cup finely chopped tomatoes
- 1/4 cup of leaf spinach
- 1 tsp olive oil - Salt and pepper to taste

How to Prepare:
1. Beat the eggs in a bowl until thoroughly blended. Add pepper and salt for seasoning.
2. In a nonstick skillet, warm the olive oil over medium heat.
3. Add the chopped veggies to the skillet and cook them until they become soft.
4. Transfer the whisked eggs onto the veggies, turning the pan to ensure even distribution.
5. Continue cooking until the omelet is set and has a golden brown bottom.
6. When serving hot, fold the omelet in half.

Time Required for Preparation: 10 minutes

Nutritional Worth (per Serving): About 200 calories, 12g of protein, 10g of fat, 10g of carbs, and 3g of fiber

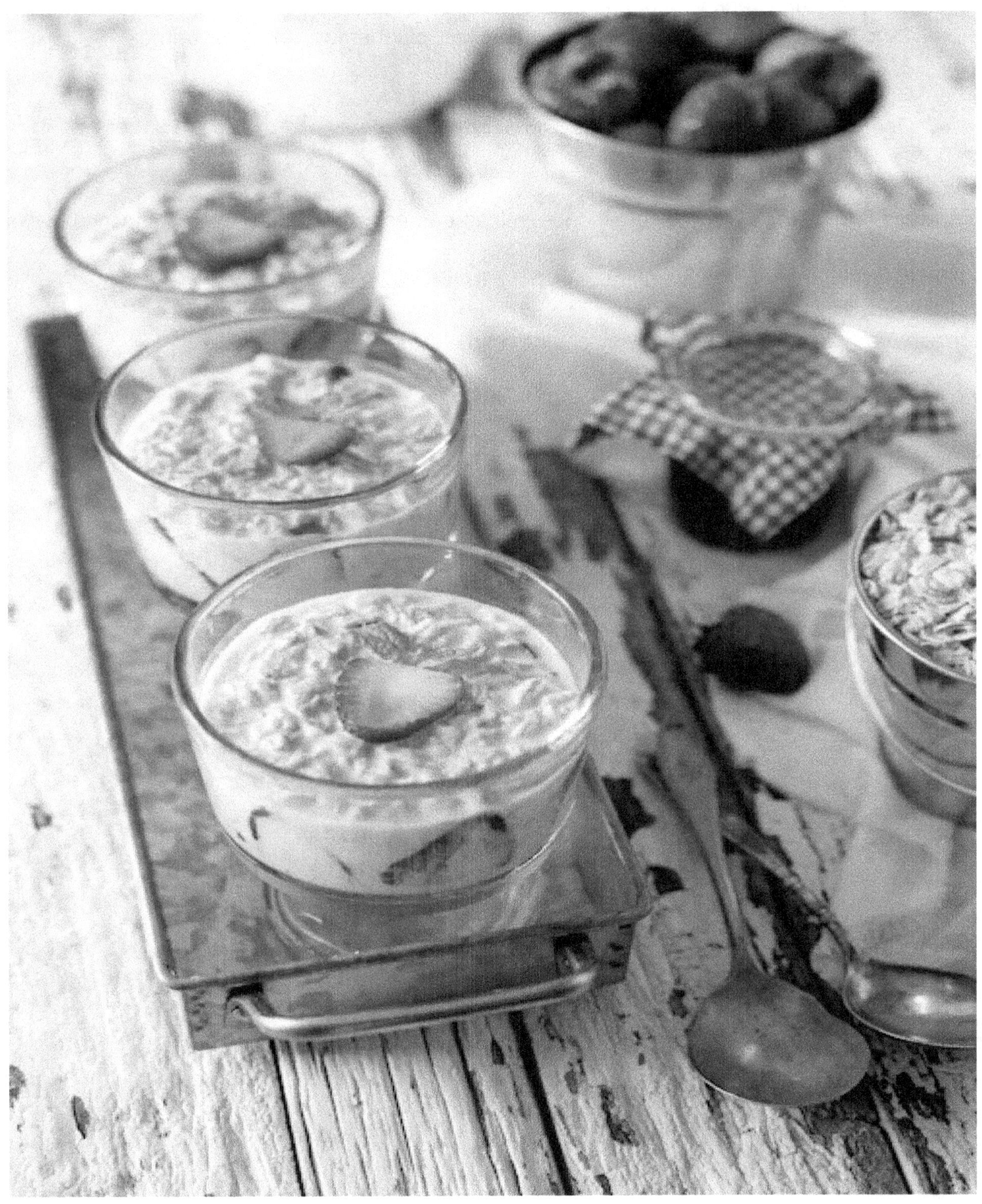

Components:

- One-half cup Greek yogurt, plain
- 1/4 cup of mixed berries, including raspberries, blueberries, and strawberries
- 2 tablespoons chopped nuts (walnuts, almonds)
- One tablespoon of chia seeds
- One teaspoon of optional maple syrup or honey

How to Prepare:

1. Arrange Greek yogurt, chopped almonds, mixed berries, and chia seeds in a serving bowl or glass.
2. Continue layering until all the ingredients have been utilized.
3. If desired, drizzle some maple syrup or honey over top.
4. When ready to eat, serve right away or store in the refrigerator.

Time Required for Preparation:5 minutes

 Nutritional Worth (per Serving): About 250 calories, 15g fat, 12g protein, 20g carbs, and 6g fiber

3. Toast with avocado:

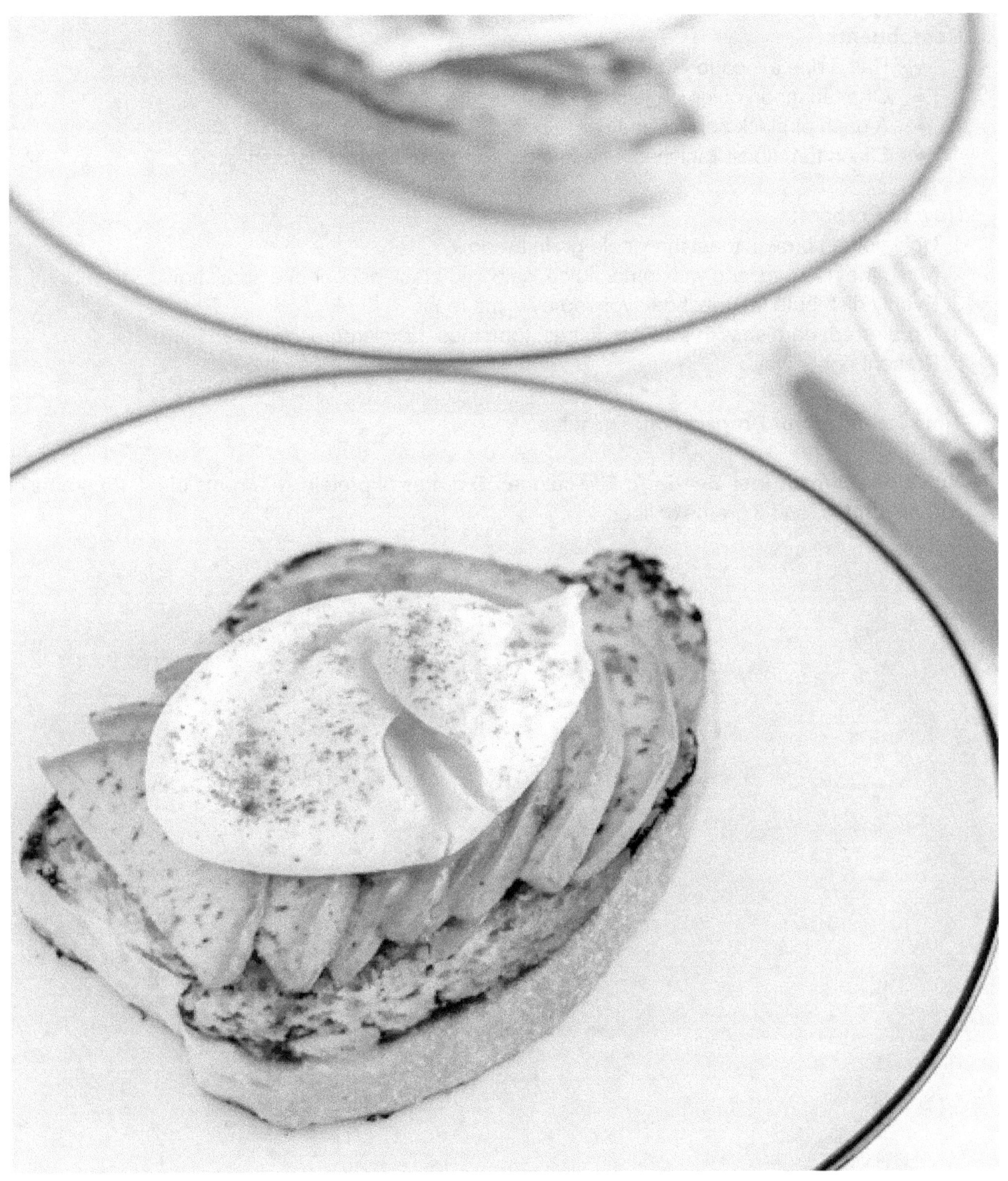

Components:
- Half a ripe avocado - One slice of whole-grain bread
- One teaspoon of lemon juice
- A dash of black pepper and salt
- Sliced tomatoes, radishes, and microgreens are optional garnishes.

How to Prepare:
1. Until golden brown, toast the whole-grain bread.
2. Mash the ripe avocado with lemon juice, salt, and black pepper in a small bowl.
3. Evenly distribute the mashed avocado over the toast.
4. If preferred, garnish with sliced radishes, tomatoes, or microgreens.
5. Present right away.

Time Required for Preparation:5 minutes

Nutritional Worth (per Serving): 200 calories, 5 grams of protein, 10 grams of fat, 25 grams of carbohydrates, and 8 grams of fiber.

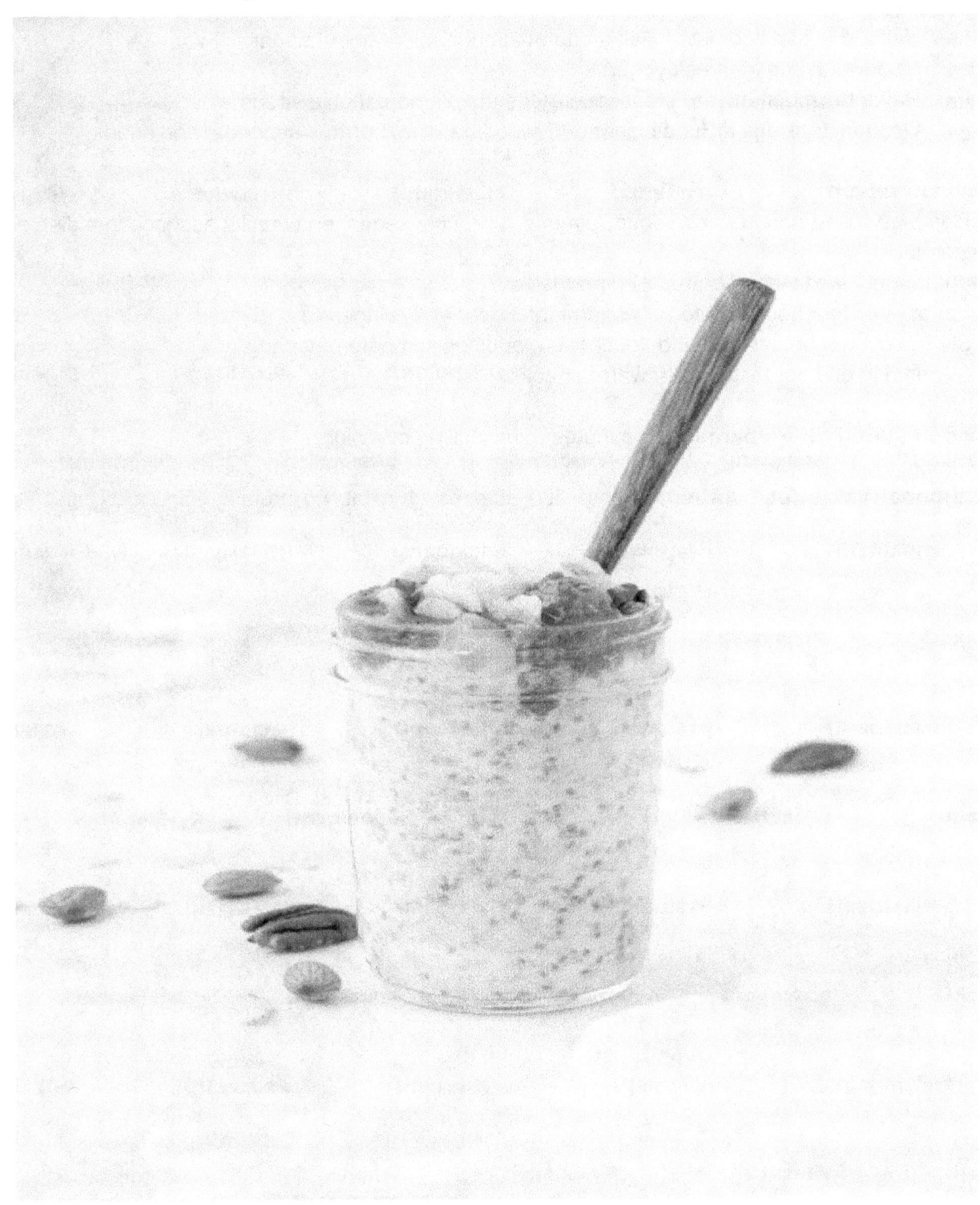

Components:

- Half a cup of rolled oats - Half a cup of almond milk without sugar
- One-fourth cup of Greek yogurt
- Half a teaspoon of vanilla essence - One tablespoon of chia seeds
- Optional toppings include cinnamon, sliced banana, berries, almonds, and seeds.

How to Prepare:

1. Combine rolled oats, Greek yogurt, almond milk, chia seeds, and vanilla essence in a dish or mason jar.
2. Thoroughly stir to incorporate all components.
3. For at least four hours, preferably overnight, cover and refrigerate.
4. Stir the overnight oats and add the chosen toppings just before serving.
5. Depending on your taste, enjoy warm or cold.

Time Required for Preparation: 5 minutes (plus chilling overnight)

Nutritional Value (per portion): About 250 calories, 10g fat, 8g protein, 35g carbs, and 8g fiber.

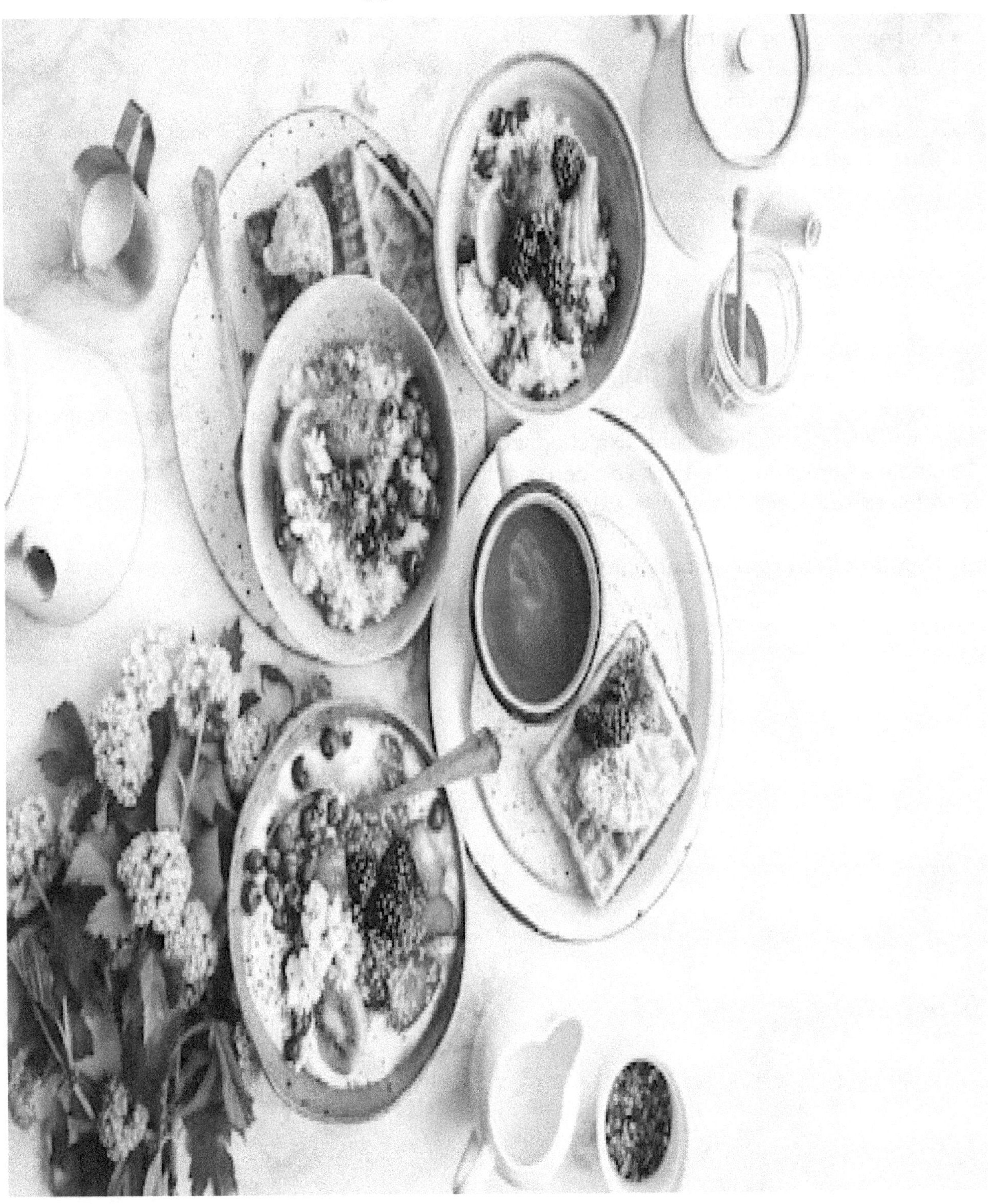

Components:

- One whole-wheat tortilla
- Two scrambled eggs
- 1/4 cup washed and drained black beans
- Two tablespoons of salsa
- 1/4 sliced avocado
- Chopped tomatoes, onions, and cilantro are optional garnishes.

How to Prepare:

1. Use a skillet or microwave to reheat the whole wheat tortilla until it is warm.
2. Fill the center of the tortilla with sliced avocado, salsa, black beans, and scrambled eggs.
3. Garnish with optional ingredients like chopped cilantro, onions, or tomatoes.
4. To create a burrito, fold the tortilla's sides over the filling.
5. If preferred, serve right away with extra salsa or hot sauce.

Time Required for Preparation: 10 minutes

Nutritional Worth (per Serving): About 300 calories, 15g fat, 12g protein, 35g carbs, and 8g fiber

6. Frittata with spinach and feta:

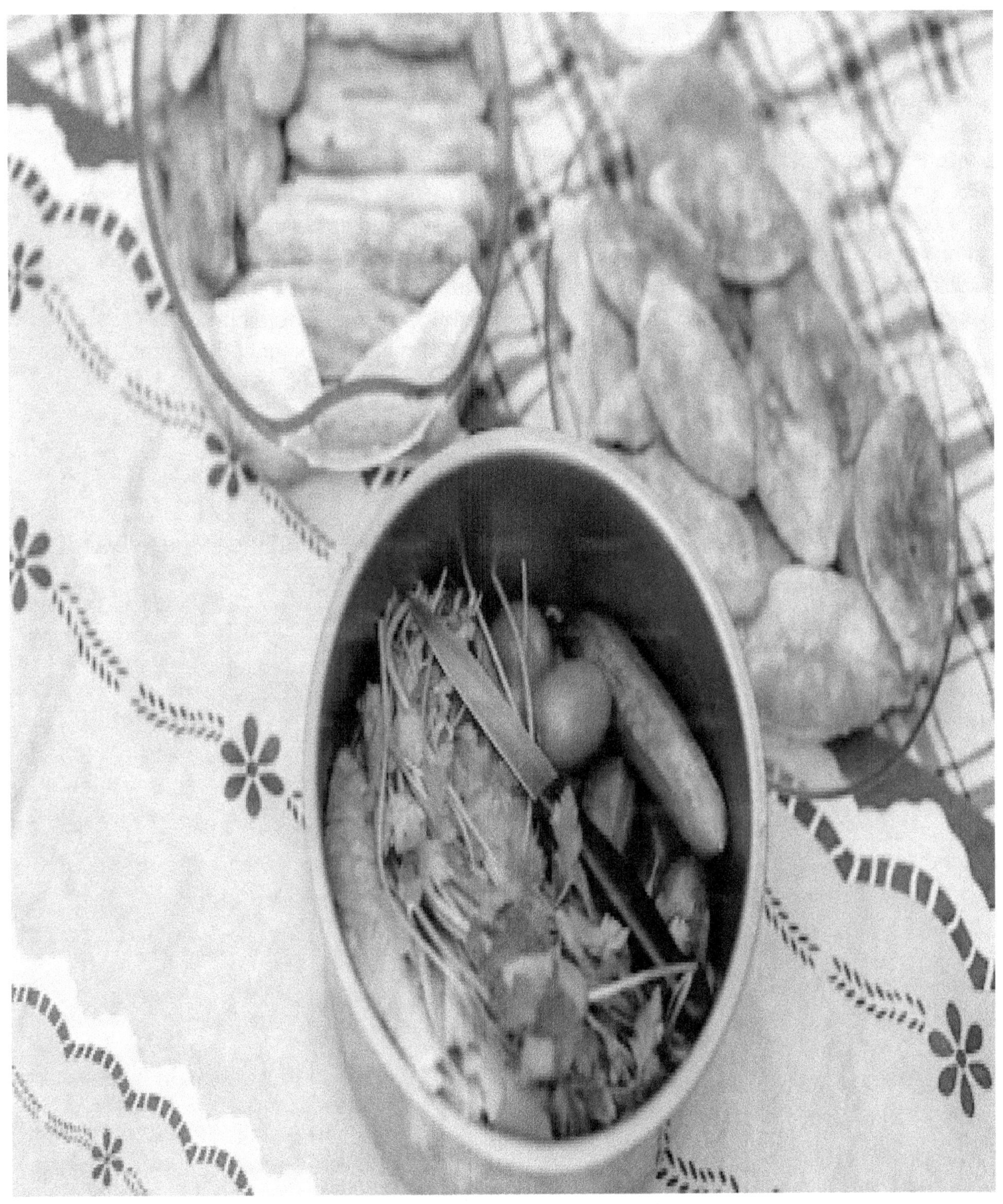

Components:
- Four eggs
- 1/4 cup almond milk or milk (without sugar) - 1 cup of fresh spinach leaves
- 1/4 cup of feta cheese, crumbled
- 1 tsp olive oil - Salt and pepper to taste

How to Prepare:
1. Set the oven's temperature to 175°C/350°F.
2. In a bowl, thoroughly whisk together eggs, milk, pepper, and salt.
3. In an oven-safe skillet, preheat the olive oil over medium heat.
4. Cook the fresh spinach leaves in the skillet until they wilt.
5. Cover the spinach with the egg mixture and top with the crumbled feta cheese.
6. Place the skillet in the oven and bake for 15 to 20 minutes, or until the frittata is cooked through and has a golden brown color.
7. Cut into wedges and warm through.

Time Required for Preparation: 20 minutes

Nutritional Worth (per portion): About 200 calories, 15g fat, 12g protein, 5g carbs, and 2g fiber

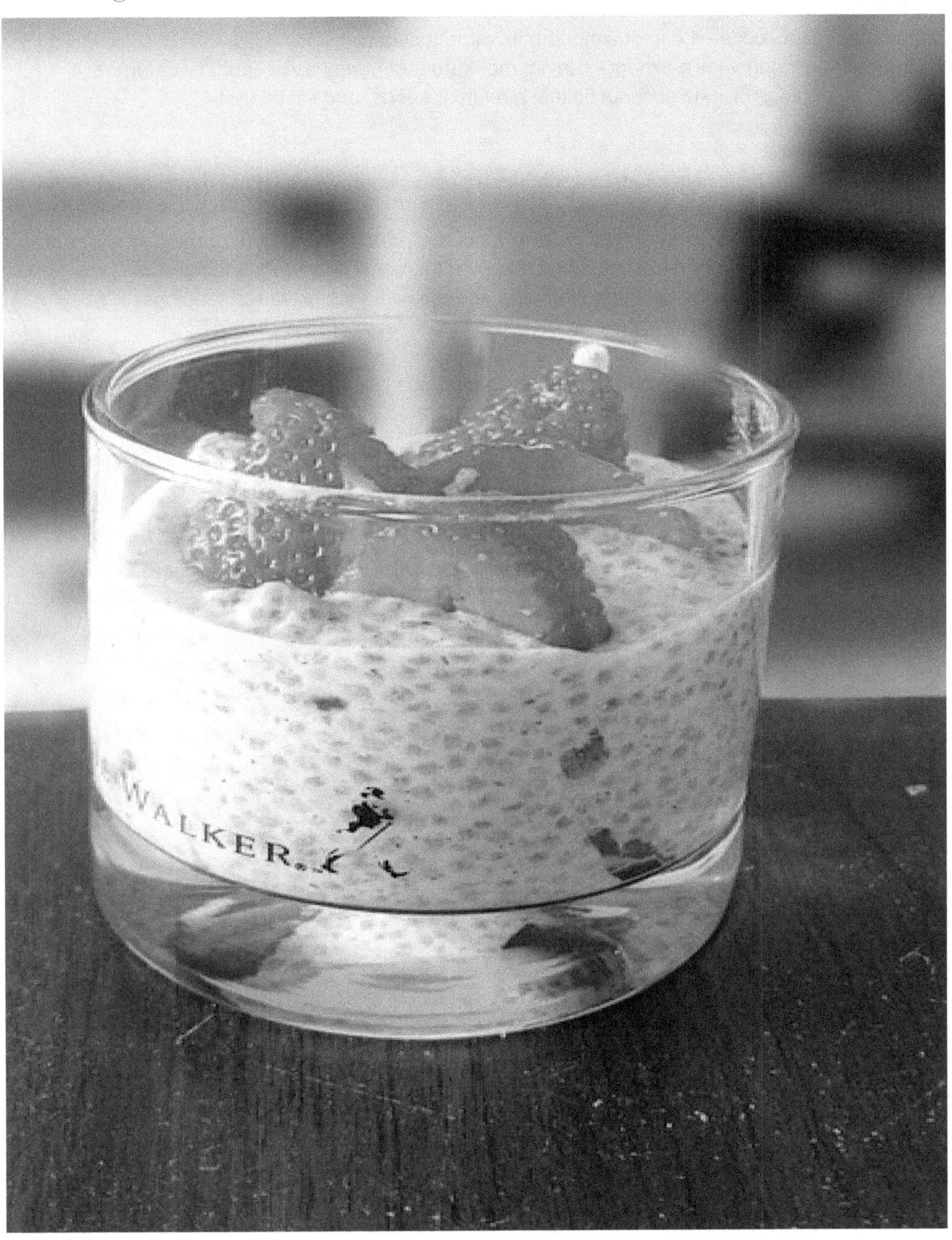

WALKER

Components:
1/4 cup of chia seeds - 1 cup of almond milk without sugar
One-half teaspoon vanilla extract - Stevia, monk fruit, or honey as optional sweeteners
Optional toppings include coconut flakes, almonds, seeds, and sliced fruit.

How to Prepare:
1. Place almond milk, chia seeds, vanilla extract, and sweetener (if using) in a bowl or container.
2. Gently stir to fully combine all ingredients.
3. Place the cover on and chill the mixture for a minimum of two hours or overnight, or until the chia seeds have absorbed the liquid and taken on the consistency of pudding.
4. Before serving, mix the chia seed pudding and top with your preferred toppings.
5. Savor chilled as a satisfying and wholesome breakfast or snack.

Time Required for Preparation: 5 minutes (including chilling)

Nutritional Worth (per portion): 150 calories, 5 grams of protein, 8 grams of fat, 15 grams of carbs, and 10 grams of fiber

8. Fruit Bowl with Cottage Cheese:

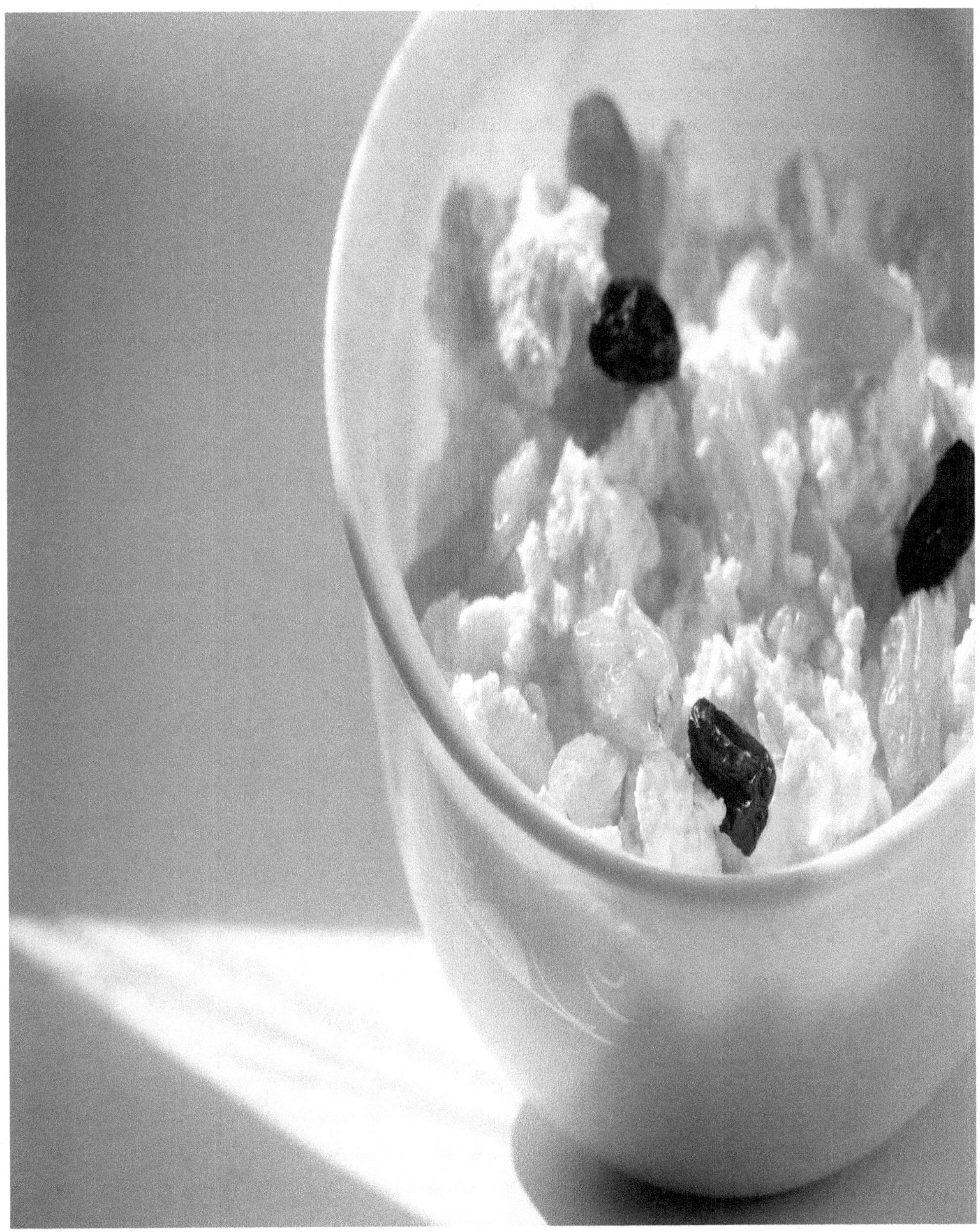

Components:

- One-half cup of reduced-fat cottage cheese
- 1/2 cup of mixed berries, including raspberries, blueberries, and strawberries
- 1/4 cup of kiwi slices
- 1/4 cup pieces of pineapple
- One tablespoon chopped nuts (walnuts, almonds)
- One teaspoon of optional maple syrup or honey

How to Prepare:

1. Arrange sliced kiwi, mixed berries, low-fat cottage cheese, and slices of pineapple in a serving bowl.
2. Add chopped nuts to the top for crunch and texture.
3. If you want to add a little sweetness to the fruit, drizzle it with honey or maple syrup.
4. Serve right away as a protein-rich and revitalizing breakfast choice.

Time Required for Preparation: 5 minutes

Nutritional Worth (per Serving): About 200 calories, 15 grams of protein, 5 grams of fat, 25 grams of carbs, and 5 grams of fiber

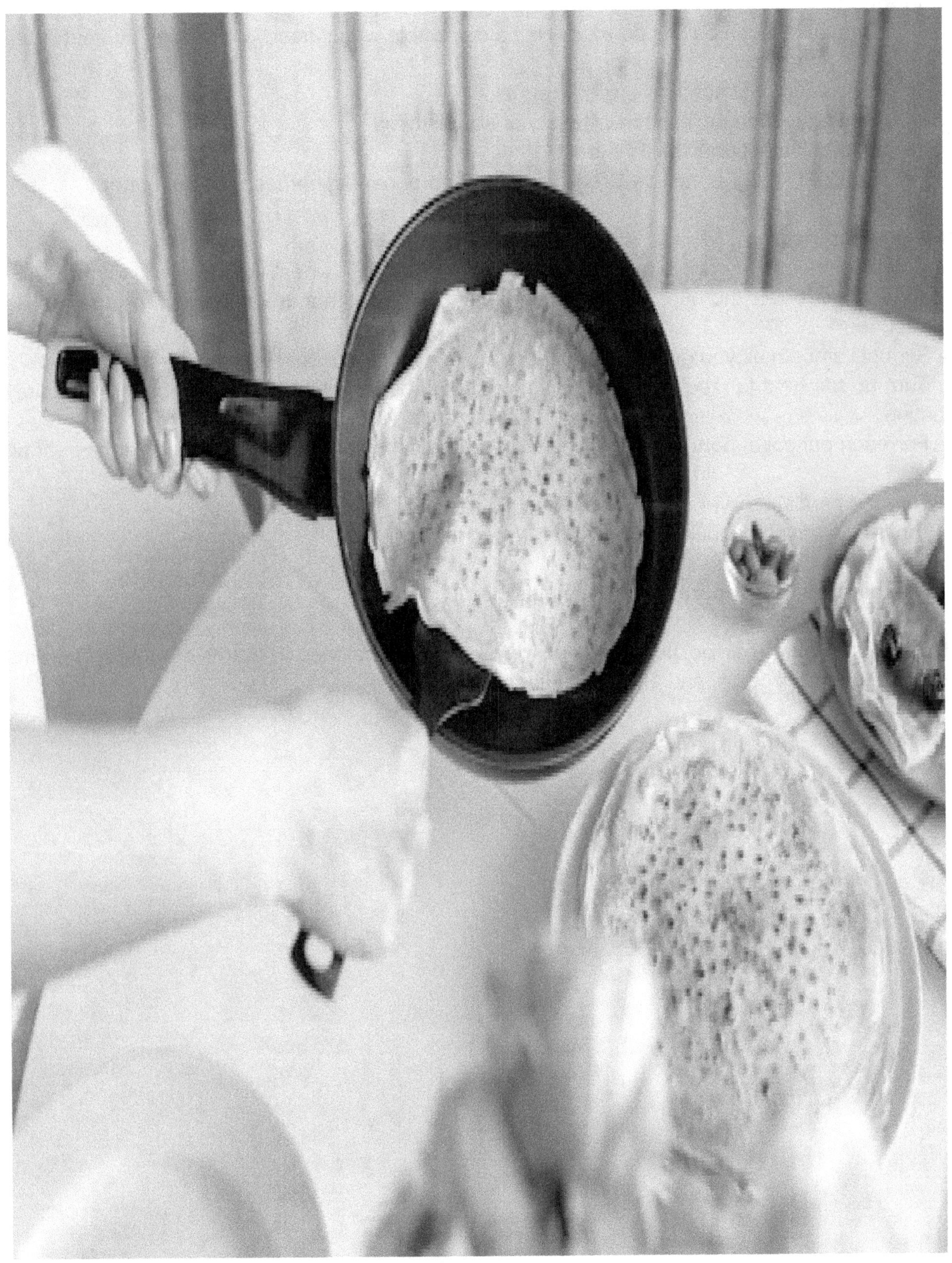

Components:
- One tablespoon baking powder - Half a cup whole wheat flour - One-fourth cup oat flour
- Half a teaspoon of cinnamon
- Half a cup of almond milk without sugar
- One egg - One tablespoon of honey or maple syrup
- One-half teaspoon vanilla extract
- Optional toppings include Greek yogurt, sliced bananas, berries, and nut butter.

How to Prepare:

1. Combine the oat flour, cinnamon, baking powder, and whole wheat flour in a mixing dish.

2. In another bowl, thoroughly mix the almond milk, egg, honey, maple syrup, and vanilla extract.

3. Stir until smooth as you gradually incorporate the wet components into the dry ingredients.

4. Turn up the heat to medium and give a non-stick skillet or griddle a quick oil or cooking spray coating.

5. For each pancake, pour 1/4 cup of batter onto the skillet and heat it until bubbles appear on top.

6. Turn the pancakes over and cook the second side until golden brown.

7. Top the steaming pancakes with your preferred toppings.

Time Required for Preparation: 20 minutes

Nutritional Value (per portion, without toppings): 150 calories, 6 grams of protein, 3 grams of fat, 25 grams of carbs, and 4 grams of fiber

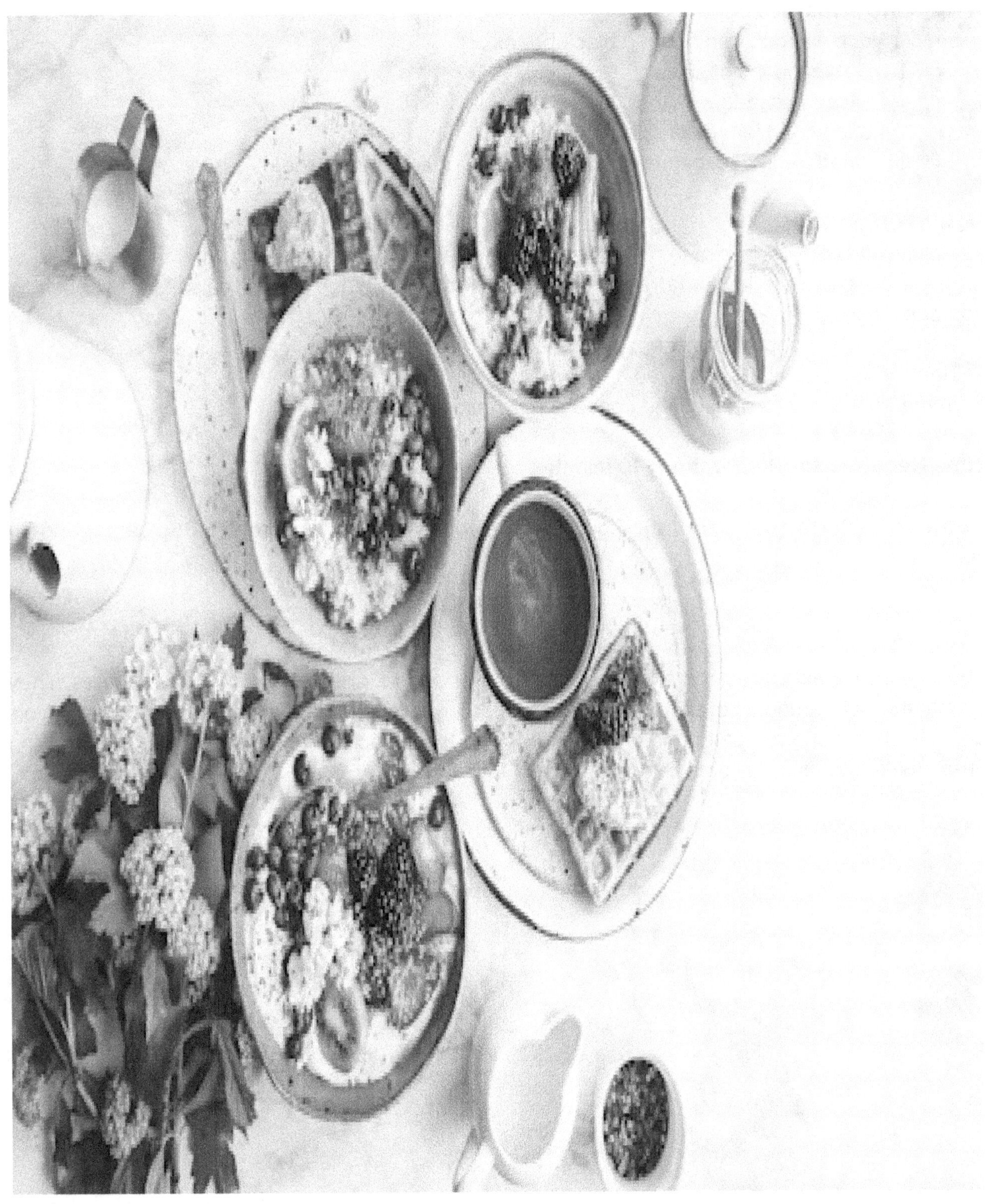

Components:

- One whole-wheat tortilla
- Two scrambled eggs
- 1/4 cup washed and drained black beans
- Two tablespoons of salsa
- 1/4 sliced avocado
- 1/4 cup young leaves of spinach
- Chopped tomatoes, onions, and cilantro are optional garnishes.

How to Prepare:

1. Use a skillet or microwave to reheat the whole wheat tortilla until it is warm.
2. In the center of the tortilla, arrange the scrambled eggs, black beans, salsa, sliced avocado, and baby spinach leaves.
3. Garnish with chopped tomatoes, onions, or cilantro, if desired.
4. Tightly roll the tortilla into a wrap.
5. Serve right away as a tasty and convenient breakfast choice.

Time Required for Preparation: 10 minutes

Nutritional Worth (per Serving): About 300 calories, 15g fat, 12g protein, 35g carbs, and 8g fiber

These easy breakfast recipes are full of nutrients and taste great for those with diabetes. They supply the right amounts of protein, carbs, and healthy fats to maintain stable blood sugar levels and advance general health and well-being. Savor these recipes as part of a hearty and filling breakfast to get your day started on the correct foot.

CHAPTER 2

GRAIN, BEANS AND LEGUMES RECIPES

1. Salad with Quinoa and Black Beans:

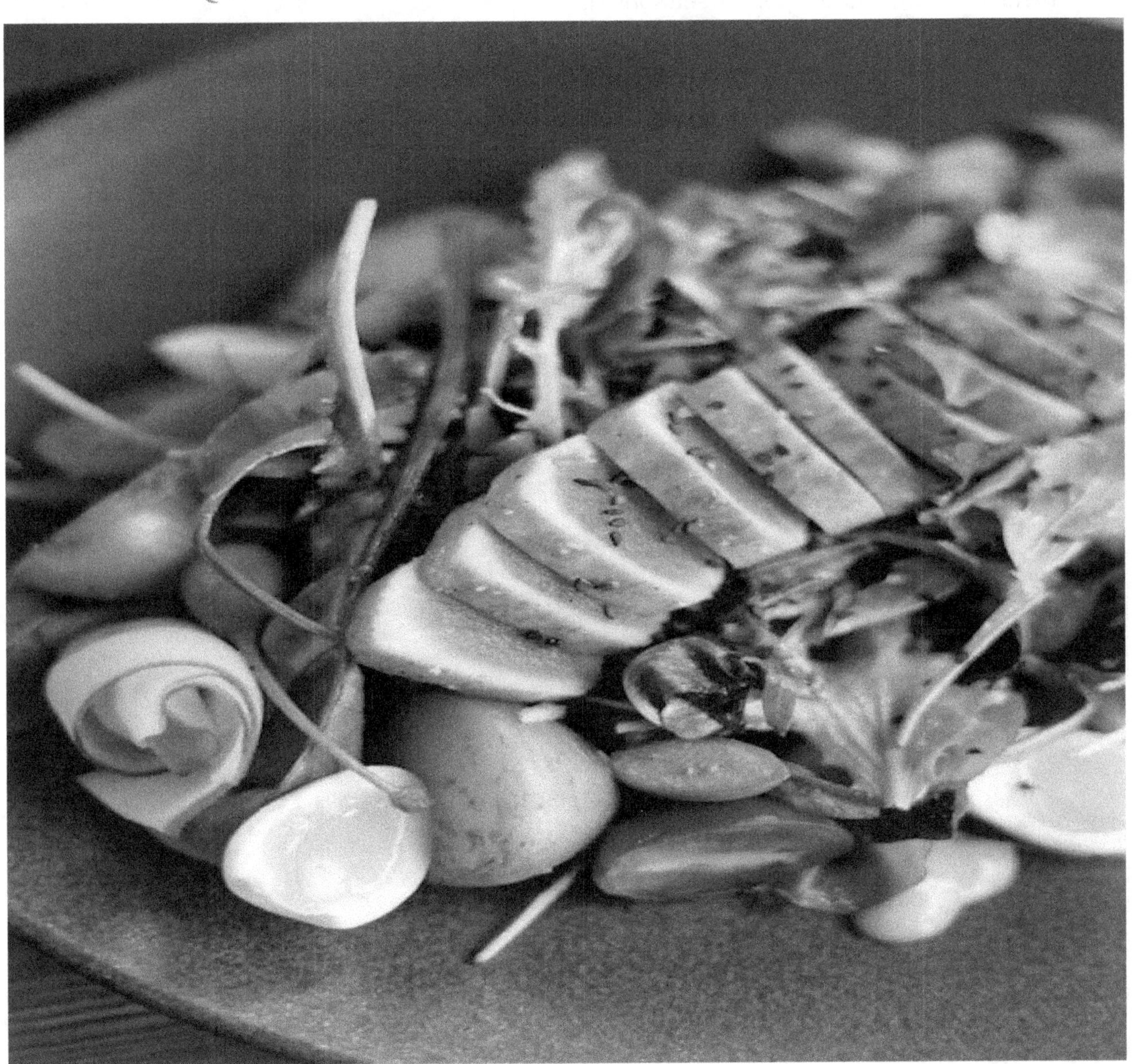

Components:
- 1/2 cup rinsed and drained black beans - 1 cup cooked quinoa
- 1/4 cup of bell peppers, chopped
- 1/4 cup of cucumbers, chopped
- 1 tablespoon olive oil - 2 tablespoons freshly chopped cilantro - 1 tablespoon lime juice
- To taste, add salt and pepper.

How to Prepare:
1. Put the cooked quinoa, black beans, chopped cilantro, diced bell peppers, and cucumbers in a big mixing basin.
2. Pour lime juice and olive oil over the salad, gently tossing to coat.
3. To taste, add salt and pepper for seasoning.
4. Serve cold as a wholesome and revitalizing salad substitute.

Time Required for Preparation: 15 minutes (if quinoa is already cooked)

Nutritional Worth (per portion): About 250 calories, 35 grams of carbs, 9 grams of protein, 8 grams of fat, and 8 grams of fiber.

2. Vegetable Lentil Soup:

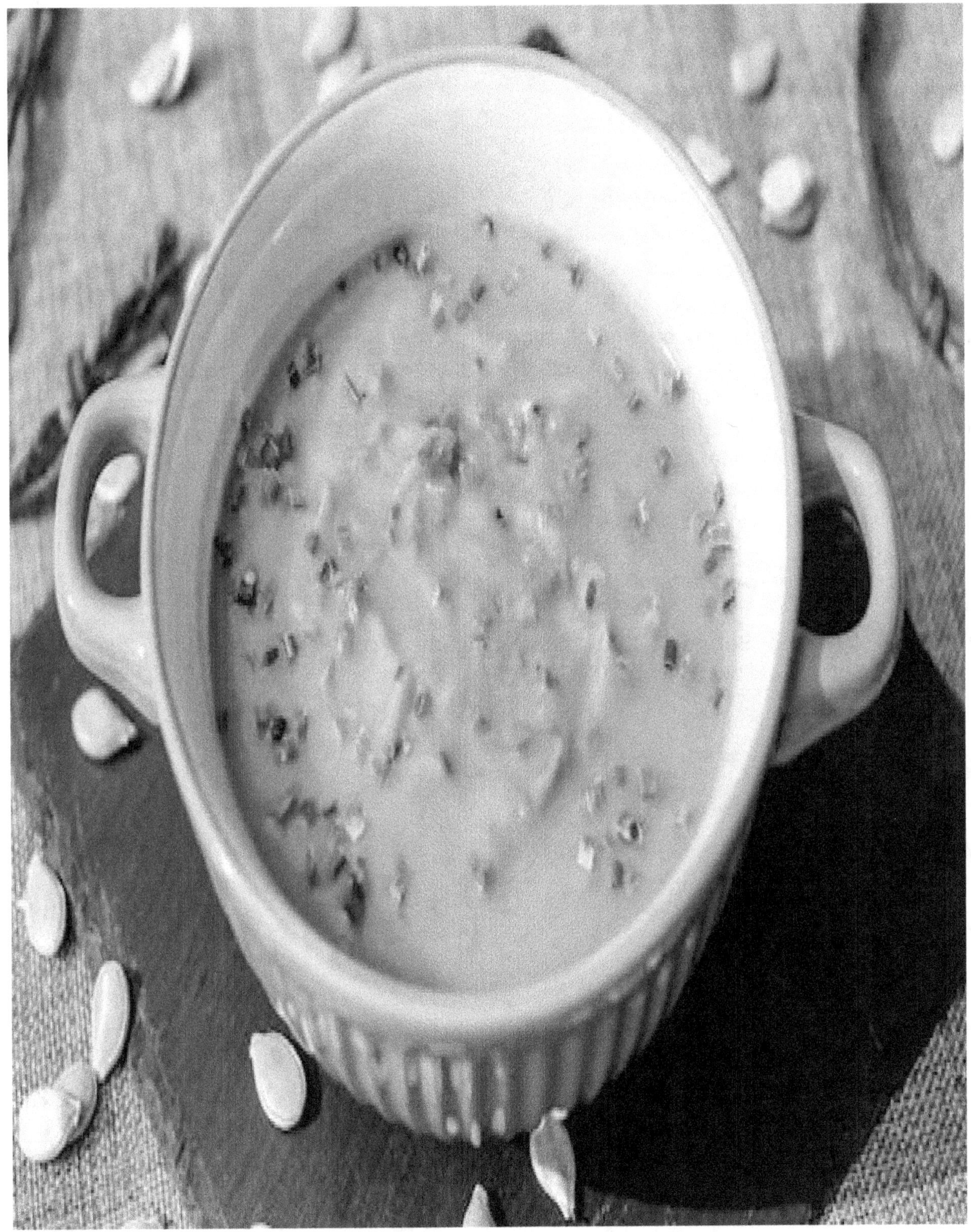

Components:

One cup of washed and drained dried lentils
4 cups vegetable broth - 1 chopped onion - 2 chopped carrots - 2 chopped celery stalks
Two minced garlic cloves
One teaspoon of dried thyme
Two tablespoons of olive oil;
 Salt and pepper to taste
To garnish, fresh parsley

How to prepare:

1. Heat the olive oil in a big pot over medium heat.
2. Add the diced celery, carrots, and onion to the pot and sauté them until they become tender.
3. Cook for a further minute after adding the minced garlic and dried thyme.
4. Fill the pot with the vegetable stock and dried lentils. Once the lentils are cooked, simmer for 20 to 25 minutes on low heat after bringing to a boil.
5. To taste, add salt and pepper for seasoning.
6. Garnish with fresh parsley and serve hot.

Time Required for Preparation: 40 minutes

 Nutritional Value (per Serving): 200 calories, 12 grams of protein, 6 grams of fat, 30 grams of carbs, and 10 grams of fiber

3. Curry with chickpeas and spinach:

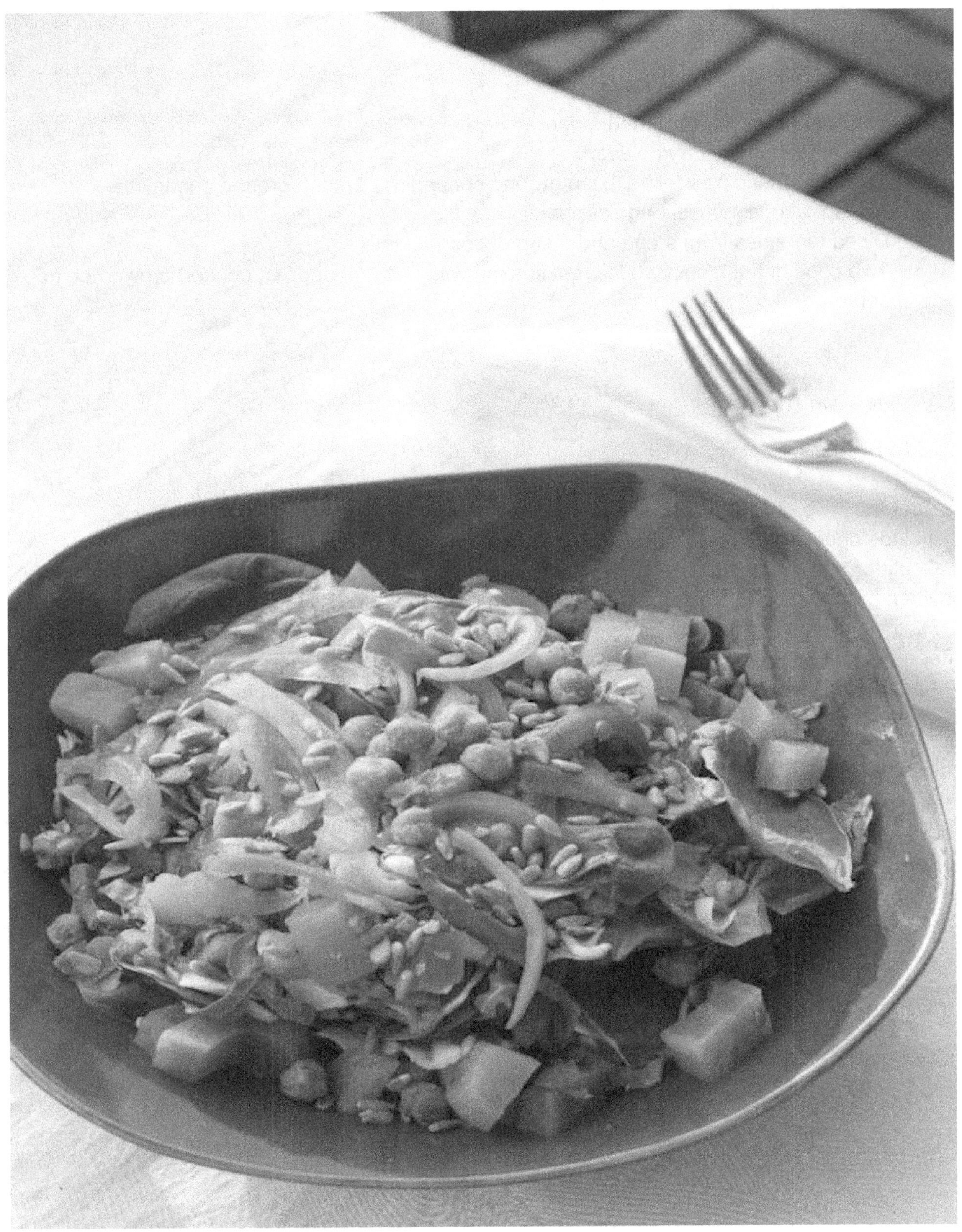

Components:

- One can of rinsed and drained chickpeas;
- - One chopped onion;
- - Two minced garlic cloves;
- - A one-inch piece of grated ginger
- One teaspoon of curry powder
- 1/4 tsp turmeric powder - 1/2 tsp ground coriander, - 1/2 tsp ground cumin
- 1/4 tsp. of optional cayenne pepper
- Diced tomatoes from a can and a cup of coconut milk
- Two cups of fresh spinach leaves; season with salt and pepper; cooked brown rice to serve

How to Prepare:

1. Heat the olive oil in a big skillet over medium heat.
2. Include chopped onion in skillet and cook until transparent.
3. Cook for a further minute or until fragrant after adding the minced garlic, grated ginger, curry powder, ground cumin, ground coriander, turmeric powder, and cayenne pepper (if using).
4. Fill the skillet with diced tomatoes and chickpeas, together with their fluids. Simmer for ten to fifteen minutes to let the flavors combine.
5. Add the fresh spinach leaves and coconut milk, then heat until the spinach wilts.
6. To taste, add salt and pepper for seasoning.
7. Top heated brown rice with.

Time Required for Preparation: 30 Minutes.

Nutritional Worth (per portion): About 300 calories, 10g fat, 15g protein, 35g carbs, and 10g fiber

4. Stir-fried brown rice with vegetables:

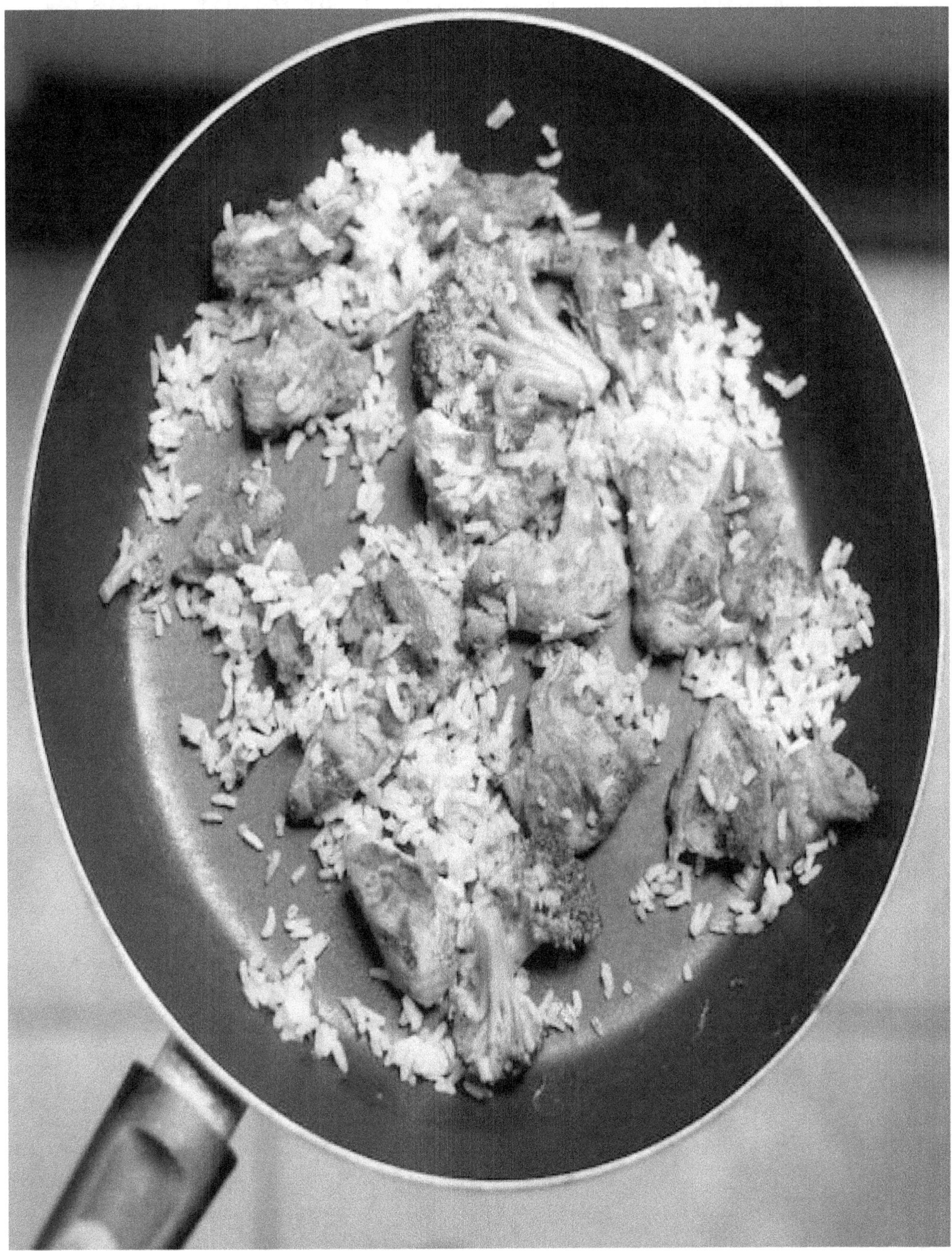

Components:

- 1/2 cup diced firm tofu - 1 cup cooked brown rice - 1 cup mixed veggies (carrots, bell peppers, broccoli, and snap peas)
- Two minced garlic cloves
- Two tablespoons of low-sodium soy sauce
- One tablespoon of sesame oil
- 1/2 tsp finely chopped ginger
- 1 chopped green onion
- 1 A garnish of sesame seeds

How to Prepare:

1. Heat the sesame oil in a wok or big skillet over medium-high heat.
2. Stir-fry the grated ginger and minced garlic in the skillet for one to two minutes, or until fragrant.
3. Fill the skillet with diced tofu and mixed vegetables. Stir-fry for 3–4 minutes, or until the tofu is gently browned and the vegetables are crisp-tender.
4. Add the low-sodium soy sauce and cooked brown rice, tossing to evenly mix all the ingredients.
5. Cook for a further two to three minutes, or until well heated.
6. Before serving, garnish with sesame seeds and chopped green onions.

Time Required for Preparation: 20 minutes (if rice is already cooked)

Nutritional Worth (per portion): About 250 calories, 10g fat, 8g protein, 35g carbs, and 6g fiber

5. Black bean and Quinoa Stuffed Bell Peppers:

Components:
- 1 cup cooked quinoa
- 4 large bell peppers, cut in half and seeded
- 1 cup washed and drained black beans
- One-half cup chopped tomatoes
- One-half cup corn kernels
- 1/4 cup of freshly chopped cilantro
- 1/2 tsp chile powder;
- 1 tsp ground cumin
- Taste and add salt and pepper as needed. Optional:
- 1/4 cup of shredded cheese

How to Prepare:
1. Turn the oven on to 375°F, or 190°C.
2. Put the cooked quinoa, black beans, diced tomatoes, chopped cilantro, diced tomatoes, ground cumin, chili powder, salt, and pepper in a big mixing bowl.
3. Thoroughly mix to incorporate all components.
4. Place the cut side up of the bell pepper halves in a baking dish.
5. Spoon the quaintly push the quinoa and black bean mixture into each bell pepper half to ensure it is filled.
6. Top each stuffed bell pepper with grated cheese, if desired.
7. Bake the baking dish in the preheated oven for 25 to 30 minutes, or until the peppers are soft, covered with aluminum foil.
8. Take off the foil and bake for a further five to ten minutes to lightly brown the tops and melt any cheese.
9. Serve hot as a filling and healthy main course.

Time Required for Preparation: 45 minutes

Nutritional Worth (per portion): About 300 calories, 10g fiber, 50g carbs, 6g protein, and 6g fat.

6. Curry with lentils and vegetables:

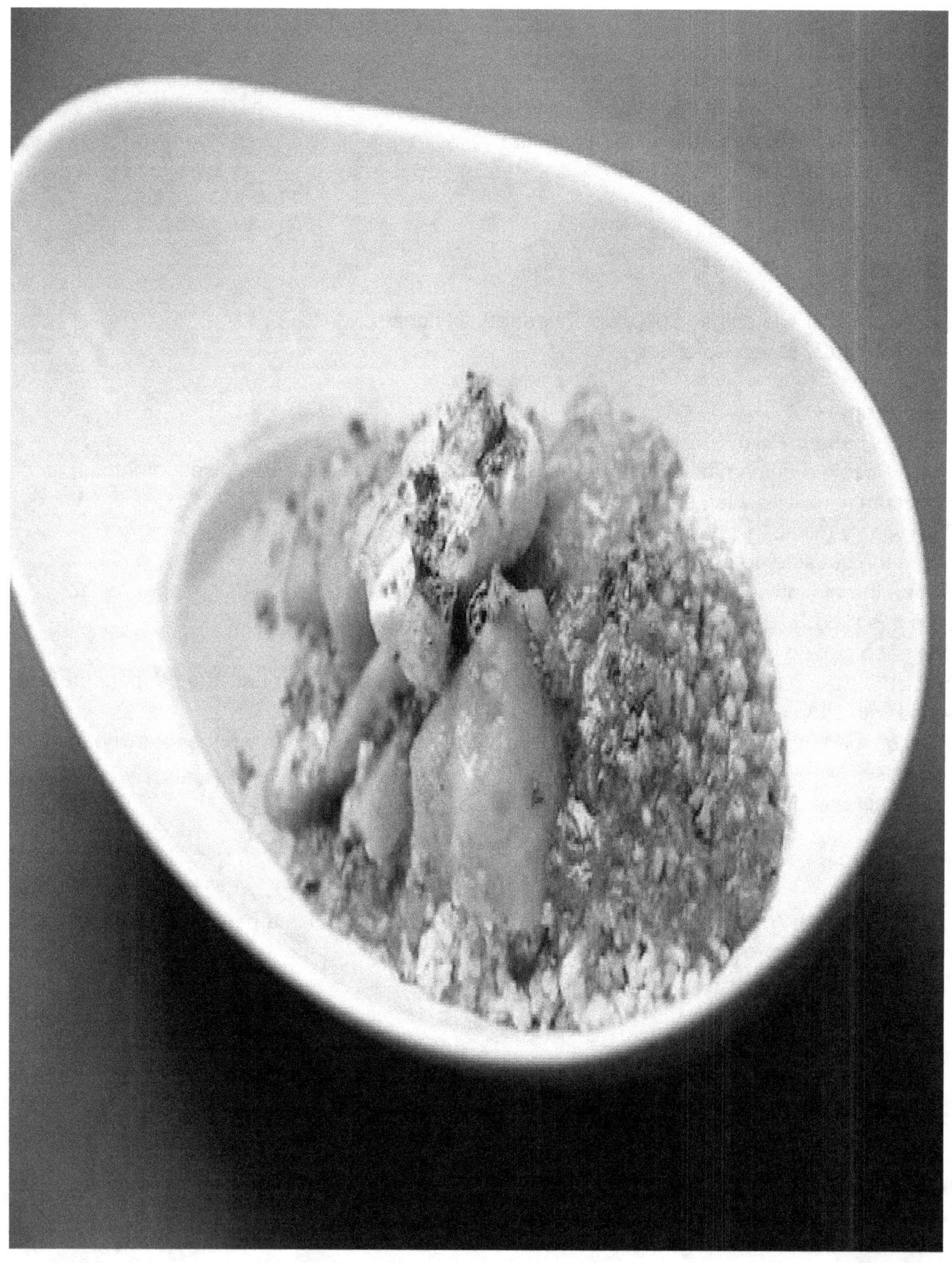

Components:
- One cup of dried lentils, rinsed and drained, either brown or green
- 4 cups veggie broth - 1 chopped onion - 2 sliced carrots
- wo diced potatoes
- One cup of florets of cauliflower
- Two minced garlic cloves
- One inch of grated ginger - One tablespoon of curry powder
- One can each of diced tomatoes and coconut milk
- Season with salt and pepper - Garnish with fresh cilantro

How to Prepare:

1. Put the vegetable broth and dried lentils in a big pot. Once the lentils are cooked, simmer for 20 to 25 minutes on low heat after bringing to a boil.

2. Heat the olive oil in a different skillet over medium heat.

3. Fill the skillet with diced onion, potatoes, carrots, and cauliflower. Vegetables should be sautéed until somewhat softened.

4. Cook for a further minute or until aromatic after adding the curry powder, grated ginger, and minced garlic.

5. Cook the diced tomatoes in the skillet for five minutes, together with their liquids.

6. Add the cooked vegetables and lentils to the pot.

7. To help the flavors combine, stir in the coconut milk and cook for a further 10 to 15 minutes.

8. To taste, add salt and pepper for seasoning.

9. Garnish with fresh cilantro and serve hot.

Time Required for Preparation: Half an hour

Nutritional Worth (per portion): About 300 calories, 10g fat, 12g protein, 45g carbs, and 10g fiber.

7. Sweet Potato and Black Bean Tacos:

Components:
- One can of washed and drained black beans
- Two cups sweet potatoes, chopped
- One chopped onion; - Two minced garlic cloves
- 1/2 tsp chile powder; 1 tsp ground cumin
- 1/4 tsp paprika smoked
- Eight tiny whole wheat tortillas - Salt and pepper to taste
- Optional garnishes include Greek yogurt, chopped tomatoes, avocado slices, shredded lettuce, salsa

How to Prepare:
Set the oven's temperature to 400°F, or 200°C.
2. Arrange the chopped sweet potatoes on a parchment paper-lined baking sheet. Season with salt and pepper and drizzle with olive oil. Roast for 20 to 25 minutes, or until soft and gently browned, in a preheated oven.
3. Heat the olive oil in a skillet over medium heat.
4. Include chopped onion in skillet and cook until it becomes transparent.
5. Add the smoked paprika, ground cumin, chili powder, and minced garlic. Cook for a further minute, or until aromatic.
6. Add the black beans to the skillet and simmer, crushing some of the beans with a fork, for five to seven minutes.
7. After roasting, add the sweet potatoes to the skillet along with the black bean mixture, stirring to blend.
8. Use a skillet or the oven to reheat whole wheat tortillas.
9. Fill each tortilla with a spoonful of the black bean and sweet potato mixture.
10. Add desired toppings, like Greek yogurt, salsa, shredded lettuce, sliced tomatoes, or avocado slices.
11. Serve warm for a tasty and filling taco alternative.

Time Required for Preparation: 45 minutes

Nutritional Worth (per portion): 250 calories, 8 grams of protein, 5 grams of fat, 40 grams of carbs, and 8 grams of fiber

8. Quinoa salad with a Mediterranean flair:

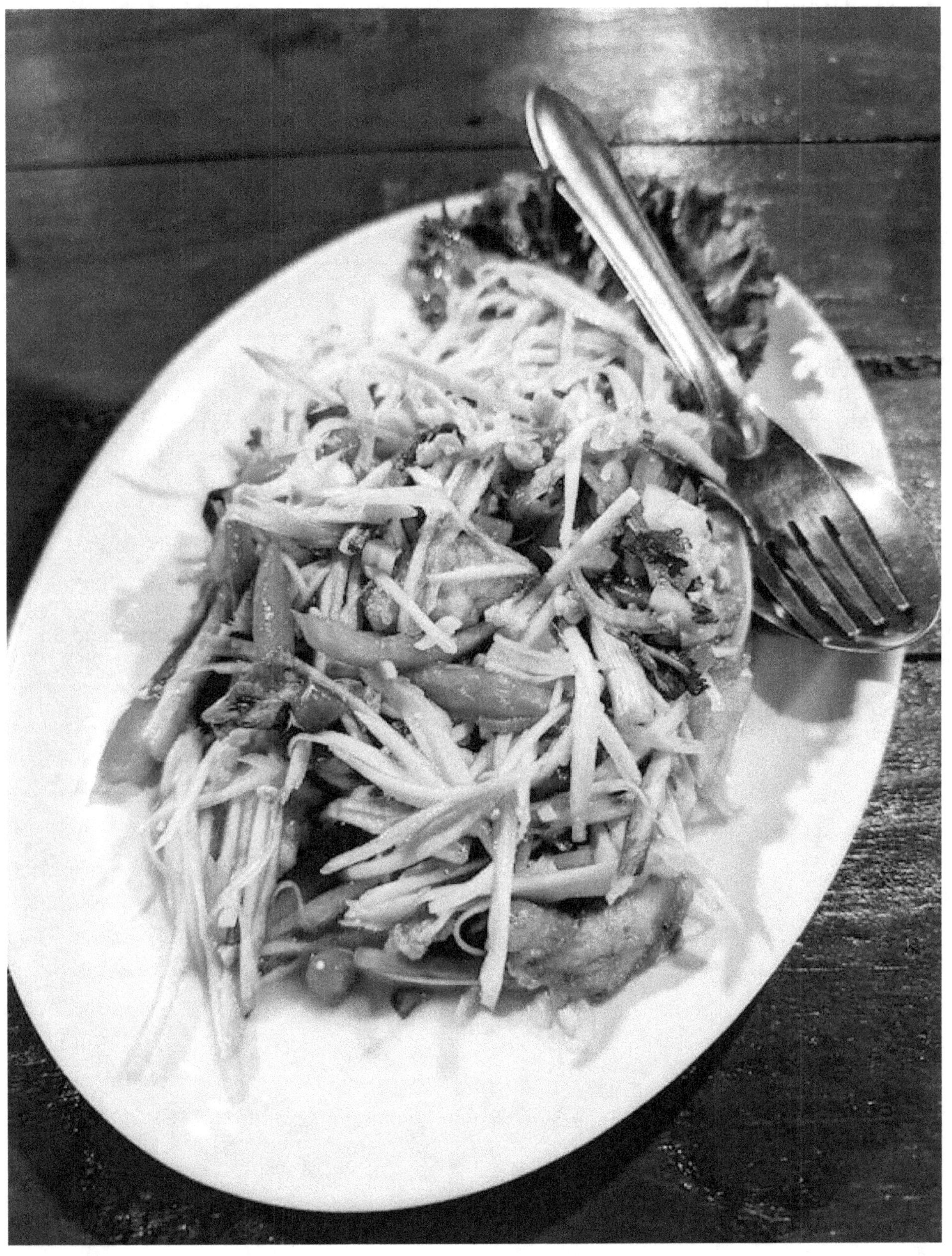

Components:

- 1 cup cooked quinoa
- 1 can rinsed and drained chickpeas
- 1 diced cucumber
- 1 diced bell pepper
- 1/4 cup diced red onion
- 1/4 cup pitted and sliced Kalamata olives
- One tablespoon of lemon juice
- Two tablespoons chopped fresh parsley
- 1/4 cup crumbled feta cheese
- Two tablespoons of olive oil
- To taste, add salt and pepper.

How to Prepare:

The cooked quinoa, chickpeas, sliced cucumber, bell pepper, red onion, Kalamata olives, crumbled feta cheese, and chopped parsley should all be combined in a big mixing dish.
2. To create the dressing, combine the olive oil, lemon juice, salt, and pepper in a small bowl.
3. Drizzle the salad components with the dressing and gently toss to coat.
4. Serve cold as a wholesome and revitalizing salad substitute.

Time Required for Preparation: 20 minutes (if quinoa is already cooked)

Nutritional Worth (per portion): About 300 calories, 10g fat, 12g protein, 40g carbs, and 8g fiber.

9. Spinach and Lentil Soup:

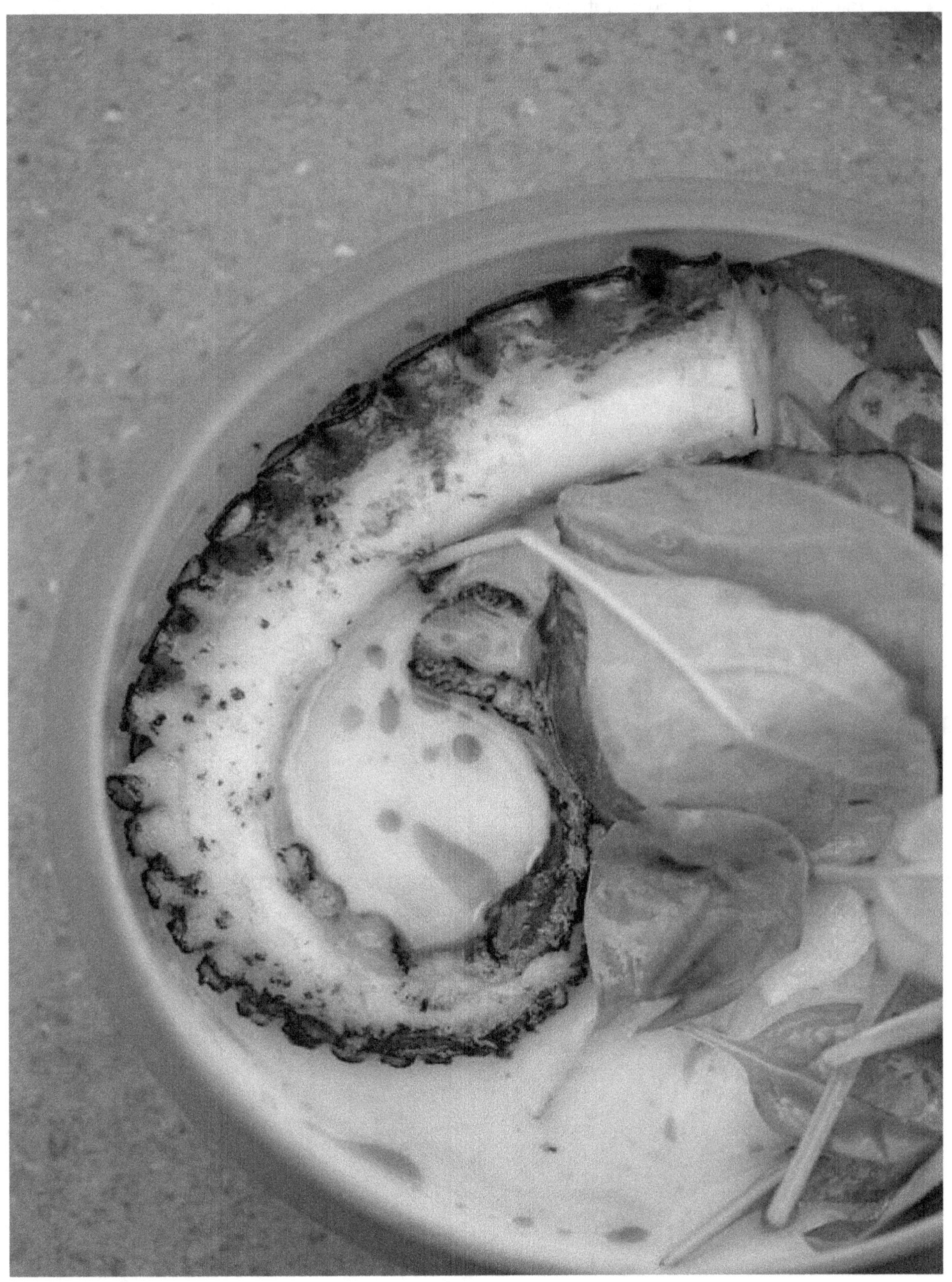

Ingredients:
- 1 cup dried green or brown lentils, rinsed and drained
- 4 cups vegetable broth
- 1 onion, diced
- 2 carrots, diced
- 2 celery stalks, diced
- 2 cups fresh spinach leaves
- 2 cloves garlic, minced
- 1 tsp dried thyme
- Salt and pepper to taste
- 1 tbsp olive oil
- Fresh parsley for garnish

Preparation Method:
1. In a large pot, heat olive oil over medium heat.
2. Add diced onion, carrots, and celery to the pot and sauté until softened.
3. Stir in minced garlic and dried thyme, and cook for another minute.
4. Add dried lentils and vegetable broth to the pot. Bring to a boil, then reduce heat and simmer for 20-25 minutes, or until lentils are tender.
5. Stir in fresh spinach leaves and cook until wilted.
6. Season with salt and pepper to taste.
7. Serve hot, garnished with fresh parsley.

Preparation Time: 40 minutes

Nutritional Value (per serving): Approximately 250 calories, 12g protein, 6g fat, 40g carbohydrates, 10g fiber

These recipes showcase the versatility and nutritional benefits of grains, beans, and legumes. They are packed with fiber, protein, vitamins, and minerals, making them excellent choices for maintaining a balanced and healthy diet, especially for individuals managing diabetes. Enjoy these delicious and nutritious dishes as part of your meals to support your overall health and well-being.

CHAPTER 3

SALAD AND VEGETABLE RECIPES

1. Quinoa and Greek Salad:

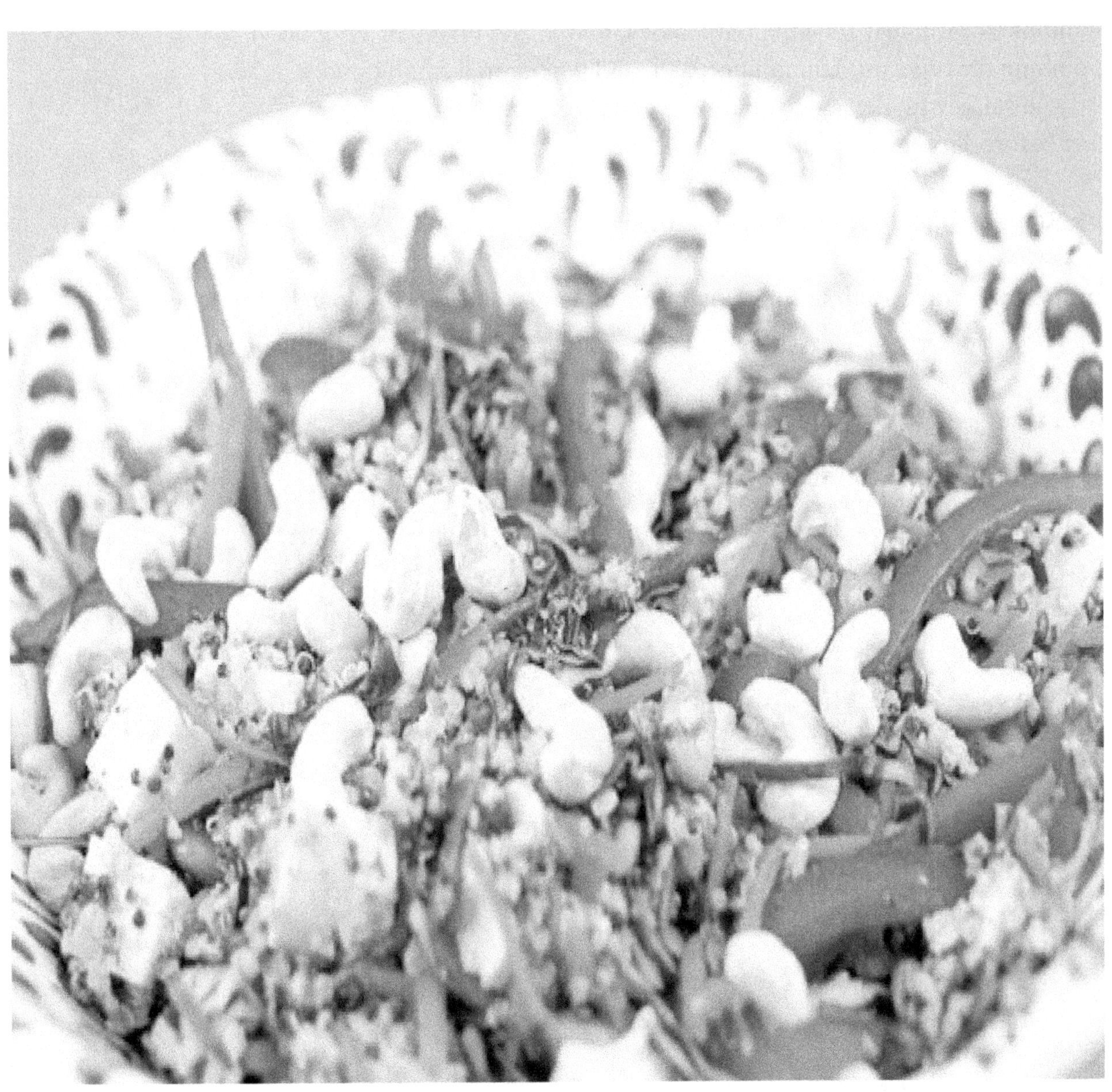

Ingredients:

- 1 cup cooked quinoa
- 1 chopped cucumber
- 1 cup halved cherry tomatoes
- 1/2 thinly sliced red onion
- 1/4 cup pitted Kalamata olives
- 2 tablespoons crumbled feta cheese
- One tablespoon lemon juice - two tablespoons olive oil
- To taste, add salt and pepper.

Method of Preparation:

1. Combine the quinoa, cucumber, tomatoes, onion, and olives in a big bowl.
2. Combine the olive oil, lemon juice, salt, and pepper in a small bowl.
3. Drizzle salad with dressing and toss to coat.
4. Just before serving, sprinkle with feta cheese.

Time Required for Preparation: 20 minutes -

Nutritional Value: Rich in fiber, vitamins, minerals, and protein. low glycemic level.

2. Asian Chickpea Salad:

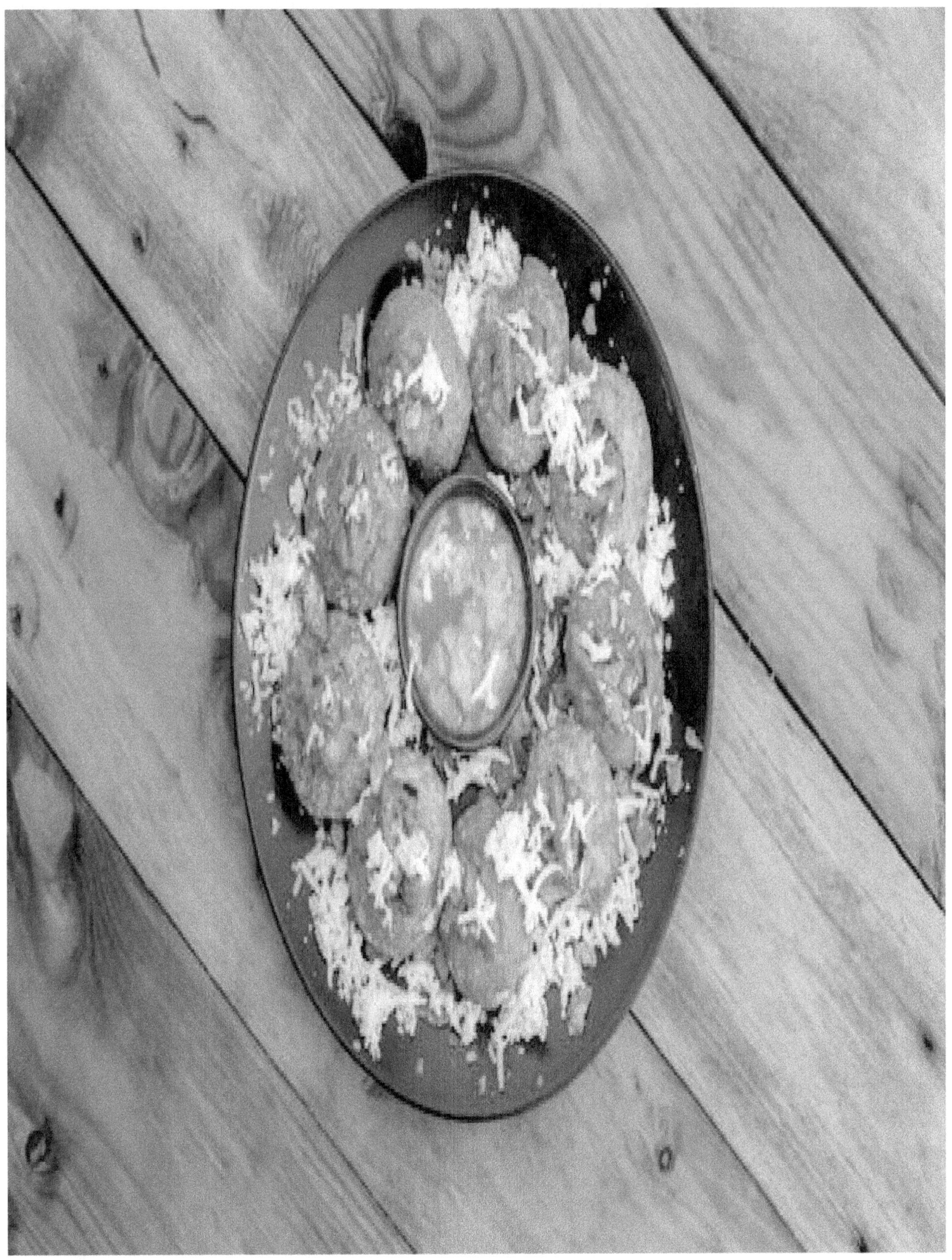

Constitution:
- 1 can rinsed and drained chickpeas
- 1 sliced cucumber
- 1 cup halved cherry tomatoes
- 1/2 finely chopped red onion
- 1/4 cup of freshly chopped parsley
- 2 tablespoons lemon juice
- One tablespoon of olive oil
- One-half teaspoon dried oregano
- To taste, add salt and pepper.

Method of Preparation:
1. Combine the chickpeas, cucumber, tomatoes, onion, and parsley in a big basin.
2. Combine the lemon juice, olive oil, oregano, salt, and pepper in a small bowl.
3. Drizzle salad with dressing and toss to mix.

Time Required for Preparation: 15 minutes

High in fiber, protein, vitamins, and minerals is the nutritional value. aids in blood sugar regulation.

3. Crunchy Vegetable Salad with Asian Infusion:

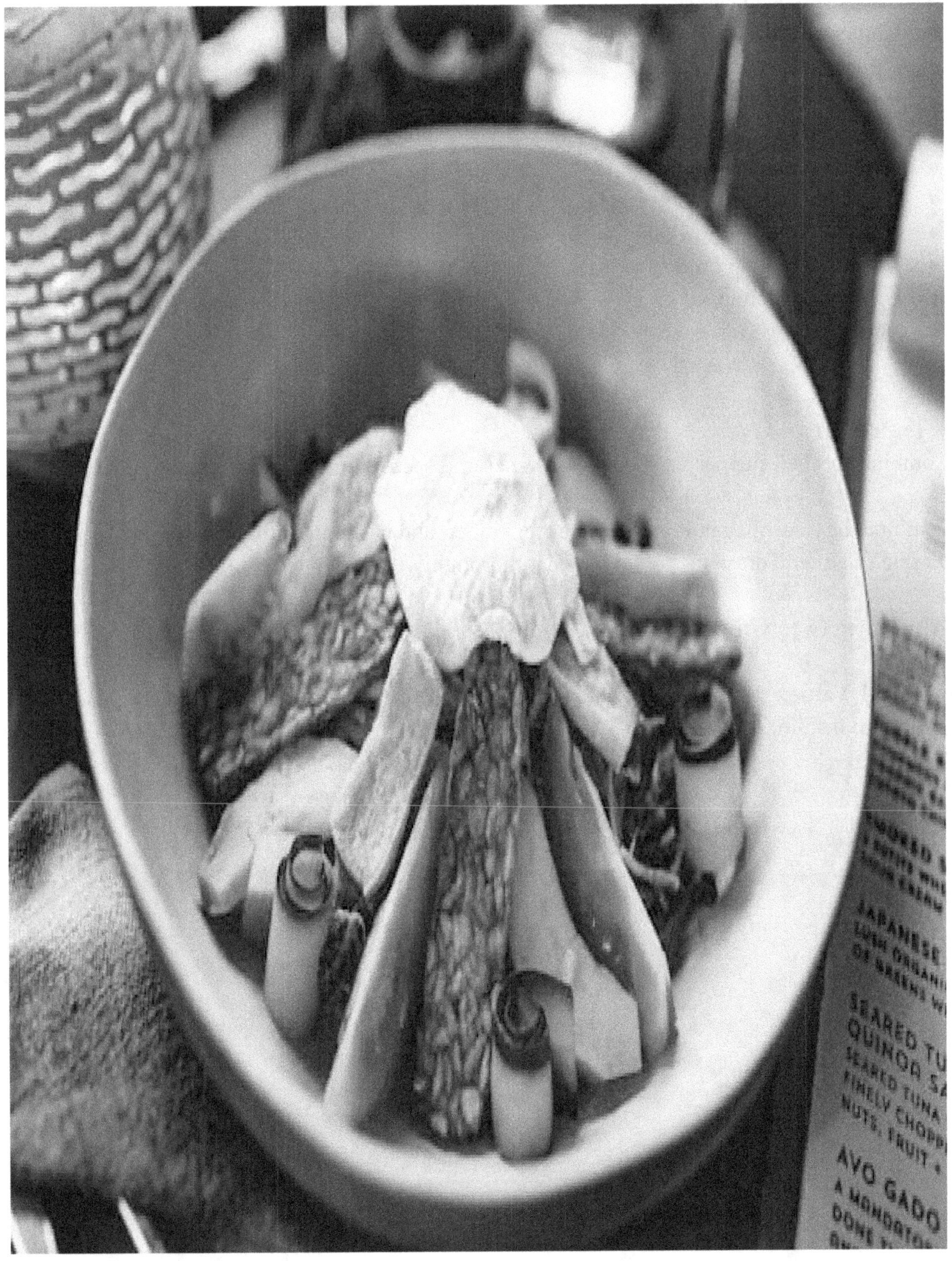

Ingredients:

- 2 cups shredded cabbage
- 1 julienned carrot
- 1 finely sliced bell pepper
- 1/4 cup of almonds, sliced
- Sesame seeds, two tablespoons
- Two green onions cut thinly
- Two tablespoons of rice vinegar
- One tablespoon of low-sodium soy sauce
- 1 tsp maple syrup or honey
- 1/2 tsp finely chopped ginger
- One minced garlic clove

How to Prepare:

1. Combine the bell pepper, cabbage, carrot, sesame seeds, almonds, and green onions in a big bowl.
2. Combine the rice vinegar, honey, soy sauce, ginger, and garlic in a small bowl.
3. Drizzle salad with dressing, tossing to coat thoroughly.

Set Up Time: Twenty-five Minutes

Nutritional Value: High in fiber, vitamins, and antioxidants, low in calories. increases one's sensitivity to insulin.

4. Vegetable Quinoa Salad with Roasted Vegetables:

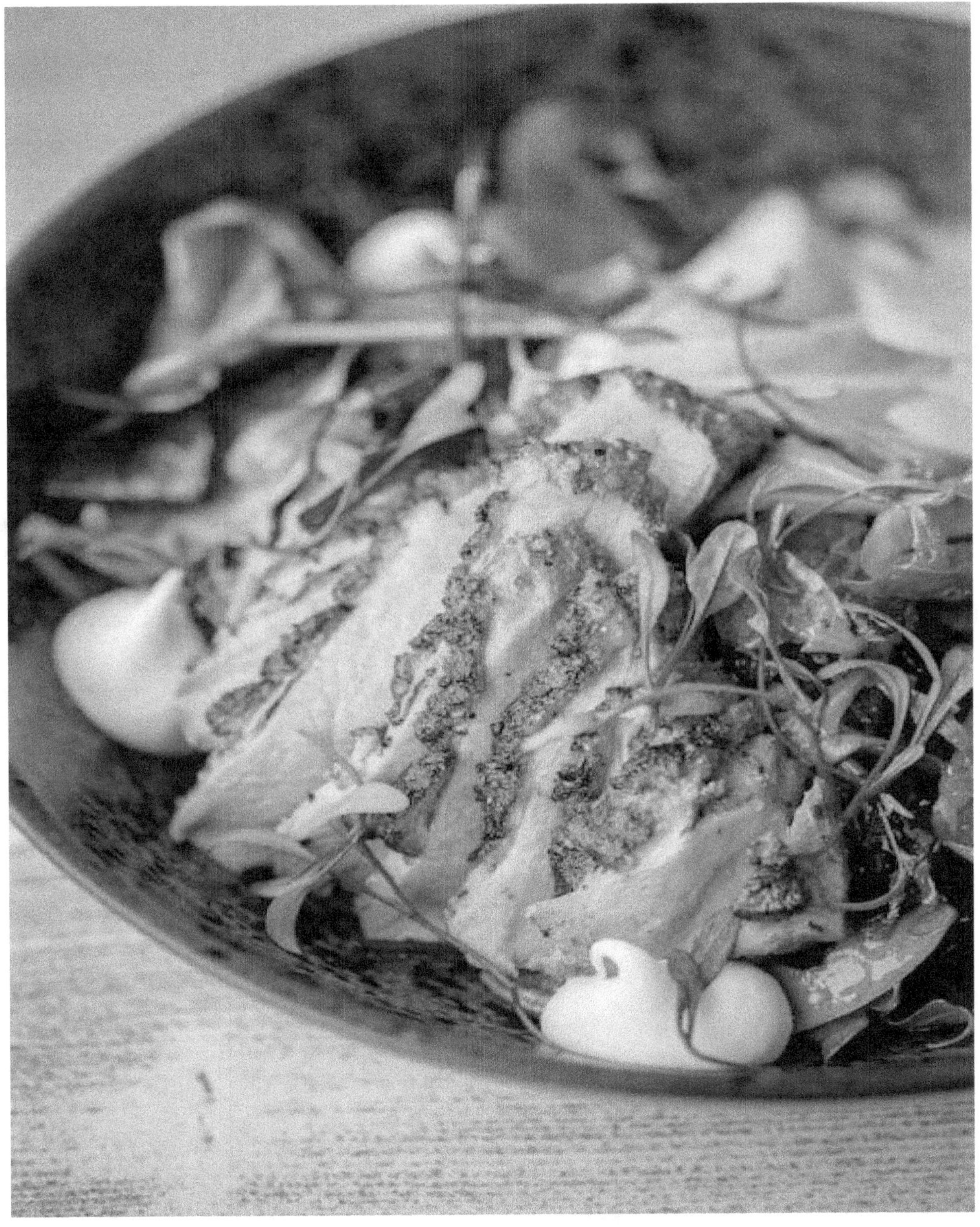

Ingredients:

- One cup of cooked quinoa
- One cup of mixed roasted vegetables (eggplant, bell peppers, zucchini, etc.)
- 2 tablespoons balsamic vinegar
- 2 cups baby spinach
- One tablespoon of olive oil
- 1/4 cup of feta cheese, crumbled (optional)
- To taste, add salt and pepper.

How to Prepare:

1. Set oven temperature to 200°C/400°F. Spread out mixed vegetables on a baking sheet after tossing them with olive oil, salt, and pepper. Roast for 20 to 25 minutes, or until soft and beginning to turn golden.
2. Combine baby spinach, roasted veggies, and cooked quinoa in a big bowl.
3. Add a balsamic vinegar drizzle and mix thoroughly.
4. If preferred, sprinkle some crumbled feta cheese on top before serving.

Time Required for Preparation: Half an hour

Nutritional Value: A well-balanced supply of protein, healthy fats, and carbohydrates. low glycemic level.

5. Poppy Seed Dressing with Spinach and Strawberry Salad:

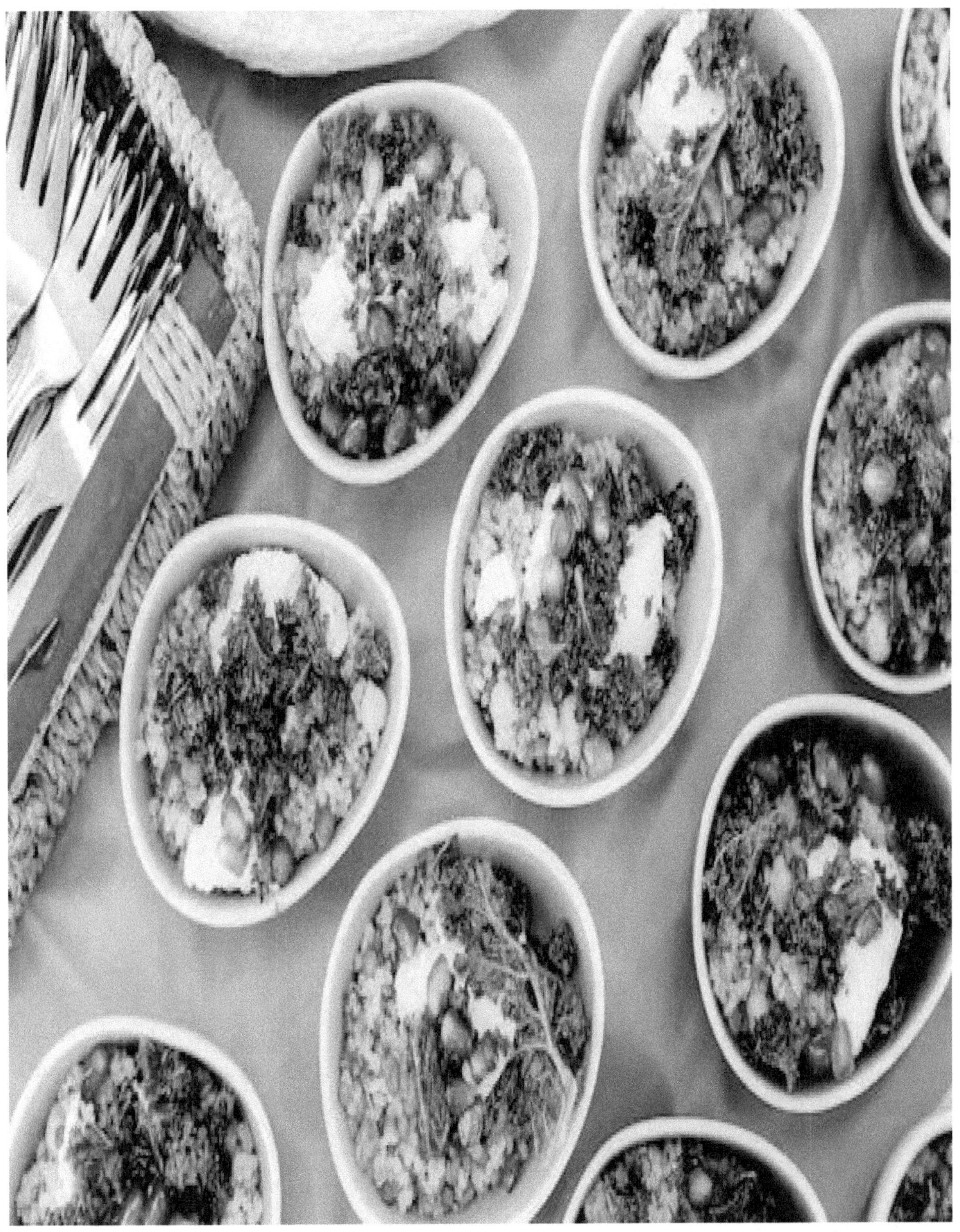

Ingredients:

- One cup of sliced strawberries
- Two cups of baby spinach
- 1/4 cup of almonds, sliced
- 2 tablespoons of crumbled goat cheese
- One tablespoon olive oil; two tablespoons balsamic vinegar; one tablespoon honey
- A half-tsp of poppy seeds
- To taste, add salt and pepper.

Method of Preparation:

1. Combine baby spinach, almond slices, strawberries, and crumbled goat cheese in a big bowl.
2. Combine the olive oil, honey, poppy seeds, balsamic vinegar, salt, and pepper in a small bowl.
3. Pour salad dressing over it and gently toss to coat.

Time Required for Preparation: 15 minutes

Value for Nutrition: Rich in fiber, antioxidants, iron, and vitamin C. helps regulate blood sugar and heart health.

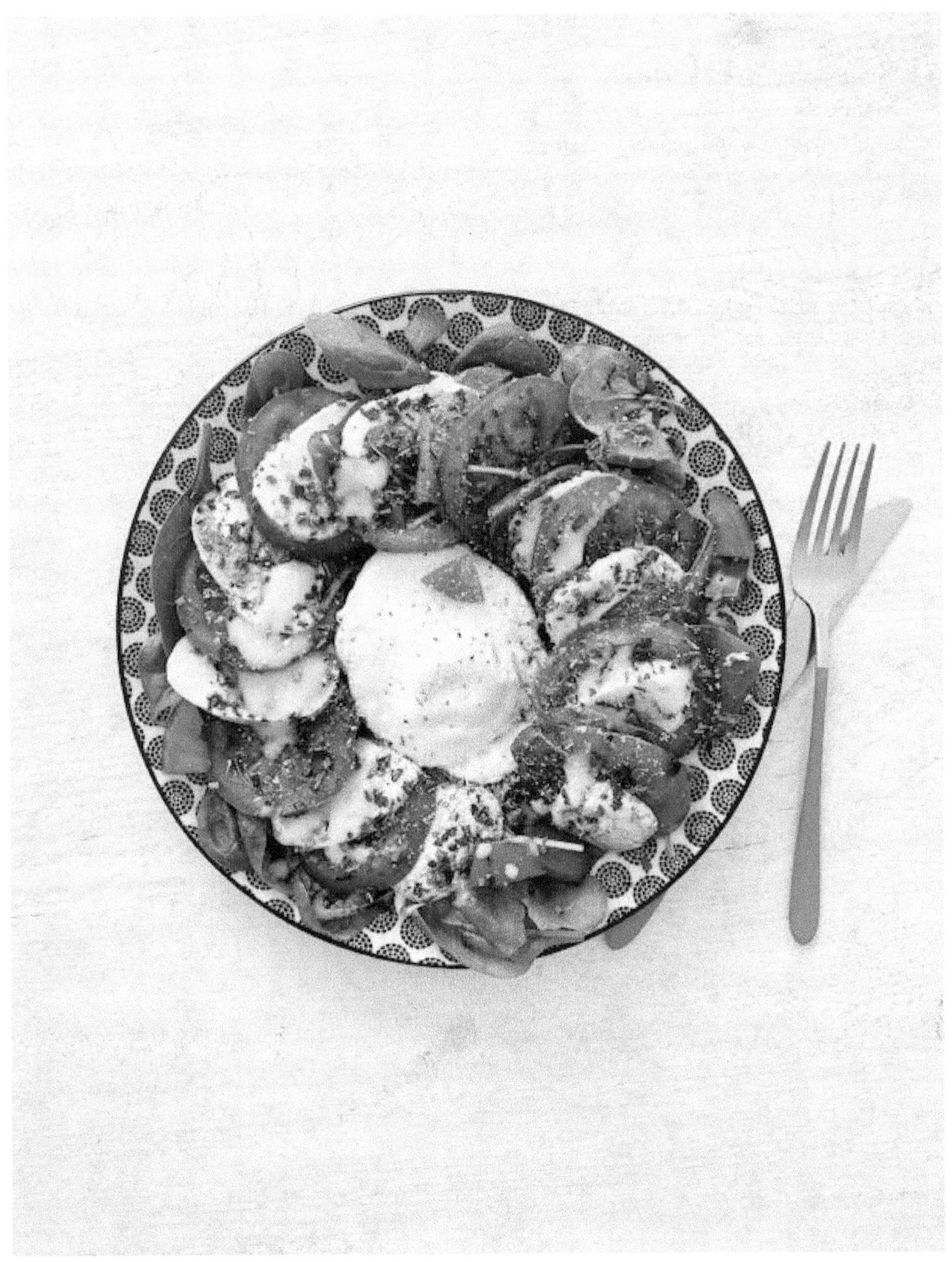

Ingredients:

- One sliced ball of fresh mozzarella cheese;
- Two ripe tomatoes
- One-fourth cup of fresh basil
- 2 tablespoons balsamic glaze.
- Adjust with salt and pepper to taste.

Method of Preparation:

1. On a serving platter, alternately arrange tomato slices, mozzarella slices, and basil leaves.
2. Season with salt and pepper and drizzle with balsamic glaze.

Time Required for Preparation: 10 minutes

Nutritional Value: **High in vitamin K and calcium, low in calories. aids in blood pressure regulation and enhances insulin sensitivity.

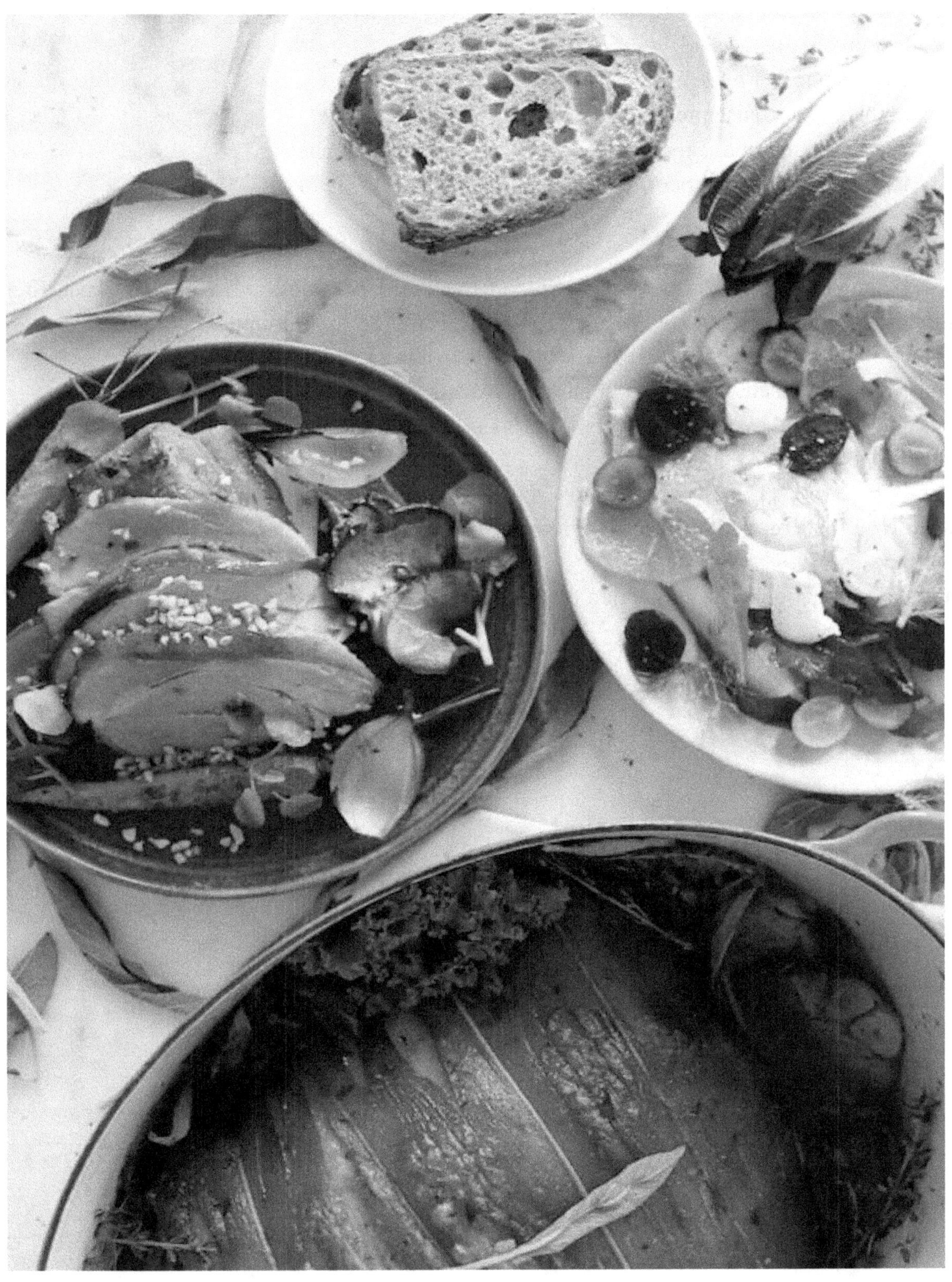

Ingredients:
- 2 medium beetroots, chopped and skinned
- 2 cups mixed green salad
- One tablespoon of olive oil;
- two tablespoons balsamic vinegar;
- one tablespoon honey; and one-fourth cup crumbled goat cheese
- To taste, add salt and pepper.

Preparation Method:

1. Set oven temperature to 200°C/400°F. Spread the diced beetroots on a baking sheet after tossing them with olive oil, salt, and pepper. Roast until soft, 25 to 30 minutes.

2. Combine mixed salad greens and roasted beetroots in a big bowl.

3. Combine the honey, salt, pepper, and balsamic vinegar in a small bowl.

4. Pour salad dressing over it and gently toss to mix. Before serving, sprinkle crumbled goat cheese over top.

Time Required for Preparation: forty minutes

Nutritional Value: Highly recommended for folate intake

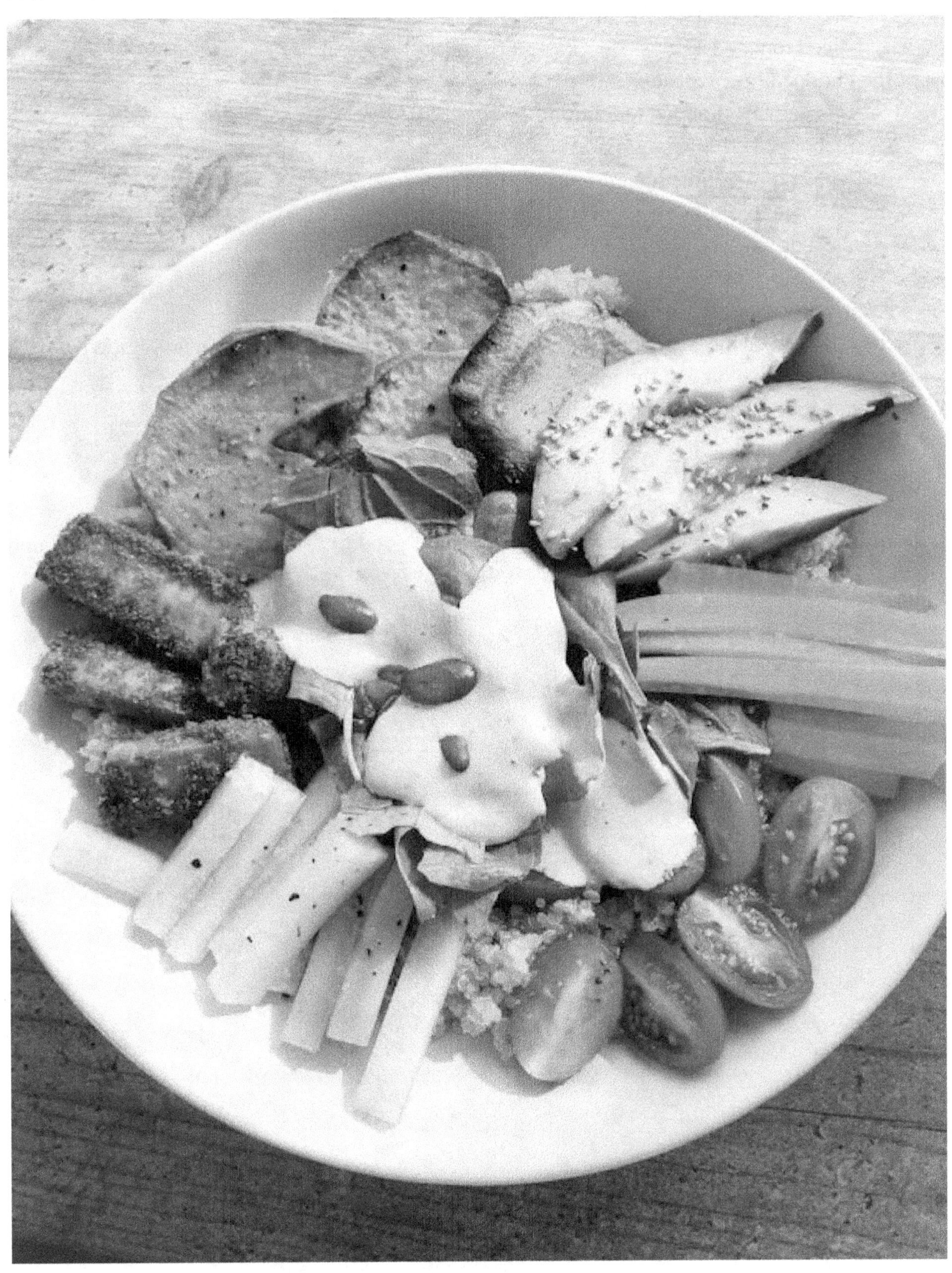

Components:

- Two diced cucumbers;
- Two diced tomatoes;
- One chopped ripe avocado
- 1/4 cup coarsely chopped red onion
- 2 tbsp chopped fresh cilantro
- One tablespoon of lime juice
- One tablespoon of olive oil
- To taste, add salt and pepper.

How to Prepare:

1. Combine chopped cucumbers, tomatoes, avocado, red onion, and cilantro in a big bowl.
2. Add a drizzle of olive oil and lime juice.
3. Add salt and pepper to taste, and toss lightly to mix.

Time Required for Preparation: 15 minutes -

Nutritional Value: Packed with antioxidants, fiber, and good fats. helps control blood sugar and heart health.

9. Salad with Broccoli and Cranberries:

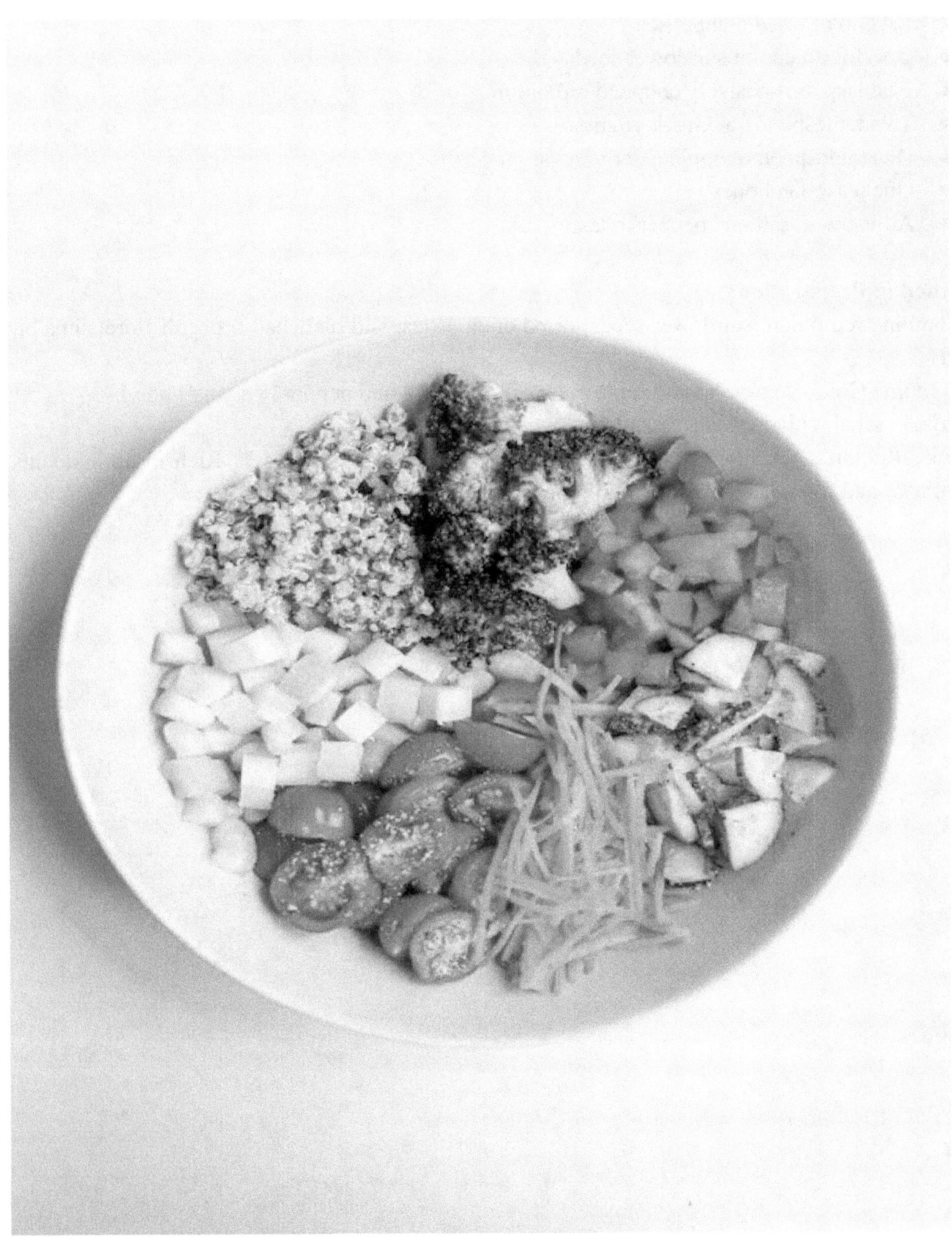

Constitution:

- 2 cups blanched broccoli florets
- 1/4 cup of dried cranberries
- One-fourth cup of sunflower seeds
- 2 tablespoons coarsely chopped red onion
- Two tablespoons of Greek yogurt
- One tablespoon of apple cider vinegar
- One teaspoon honey
- Adjust with salt and pepper to taste

.Method of Preparation:

1. Combine red onion, sunflower seeds, dried cranberries, and blanched broccoli florets in a big bowl.
2. Combine Greek yogurt, honey, apple cider vinegar, salt, and pepper in a small bowl.
3. Drizzle salad with dressing, tossing to coat evenly.

**Time Required for Preparation: 20 minutes - **Nutritional Value: ** Rich in antioxidants, vitamin C, and fiber. enhances immunological and digestive processes.

10. Lemon Vinaigrette Kale and Quinoa Salad:

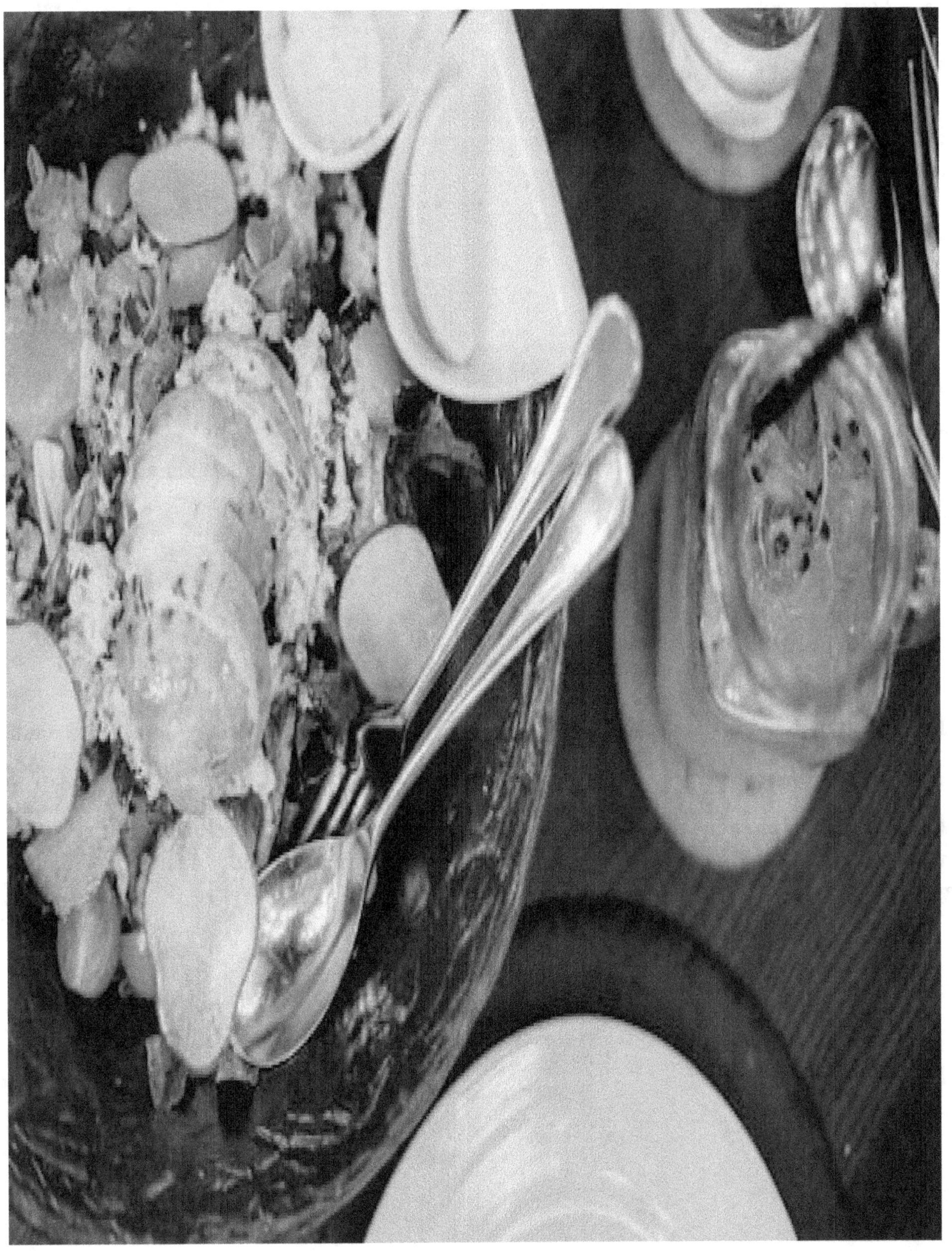

Ingredients:

- 2 cups of cooked quinoa
- 2 cups of finely chopped kale leaves
- 1/4 cup of almond slices
- 1/4 cup of cranberries, dried
- 2 tablespoons of grated Parmesan cheese
- 2 tablespoons of lemon juice
- 2 tablespoons olive oil
- 1 tsp Dijon mustard
- 1 chopped garlic clove
- To taste, add salt and pepper.
-

Method of Preparation:

1. Put the cooked quinoa, chopped kale, dried cranberries, sliced almonds, and Parmesan cheese in a big bowl.
2. Combine the lemon juice, olive oil, Dijon mustard, garlic, salt, and pepper in a small bowl.
3. Drizzle salad with dressing, tossing to coat evenly.

Set Up Time: twenty-five minutes

Value for Nutrition: rich in vitamins, protein, and fiber. helps lower inflammation and maintain the condition of the bones.

These salad dishes provide vital nutrients for managing diabetes and general health in an array of flavors and textures. Changes can be made to dietary requirements and personal preferences. Have fun trying out these tasty and healthy selections!

CHAPTER 4

<u>MEAT RECIPES</u>

1. Grilled Chicken with Herbs:

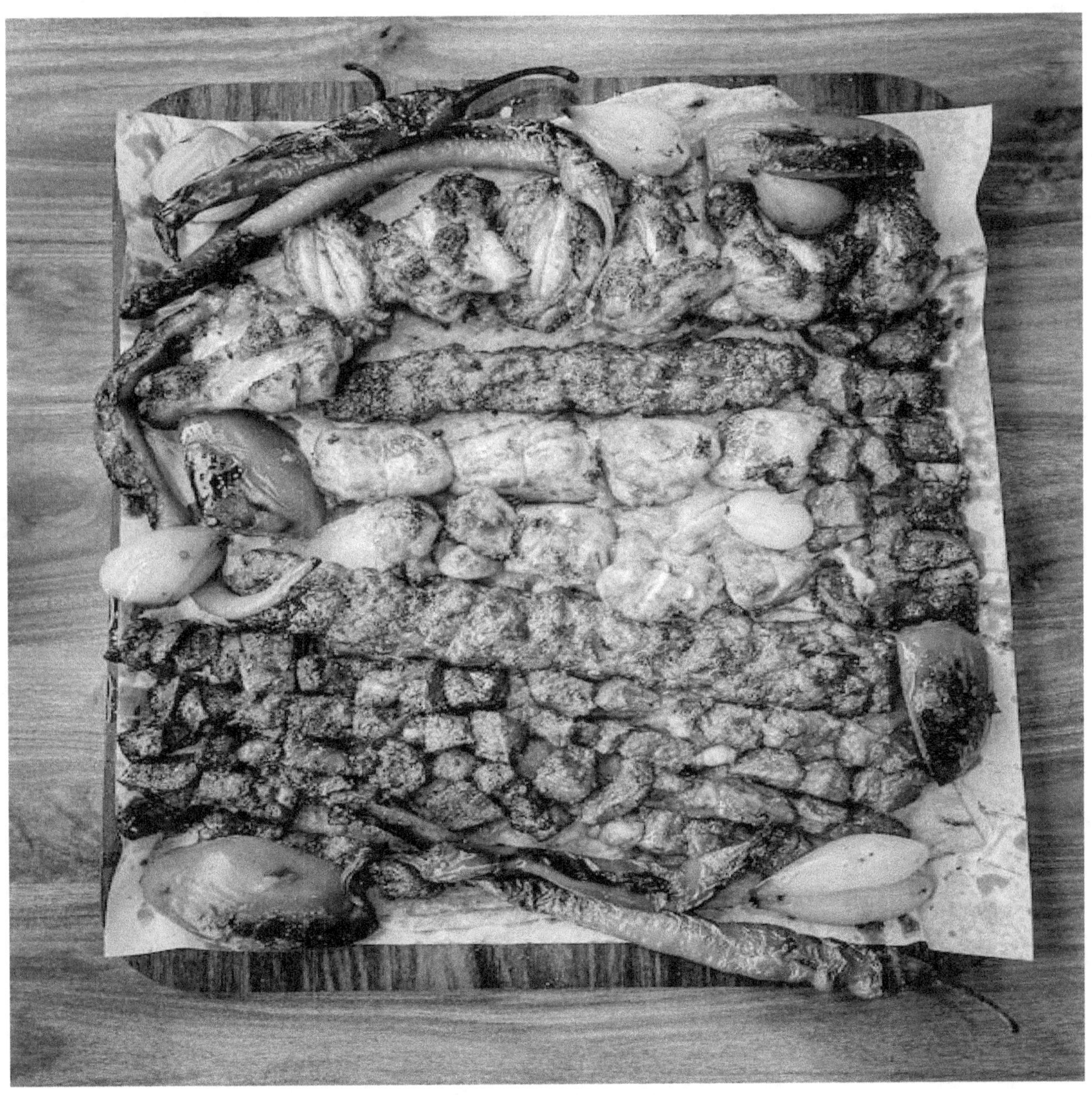

Ingredients:
- Four skinless and boneless chicken breasts
- Two tablespoons of olive oil
- Two chopped garlic cloves
- One tablespoon of freshly squeezed lemon juice
- One teaspoon of dried thyme
- One teaspoon dried oregano
- To taste, add salt and pepper.

How to Prepare:
1. Combine olive oil, lemon juice, minced garlic, thyme, oregano, salt, and pepper in a bowl.
2. Let the marinade marinate the chicken breasts for half an hour.
3. Turn the grill to medium-high and cook the chicken for 6 to 8 minutes on each side, or until it is thoroughly cooked.

Time Required for Preparation: forty minutes

Nutritional Value: Rich in protein and low in carbs, ideal for maintaining muscle mass and blood sugar regulation.

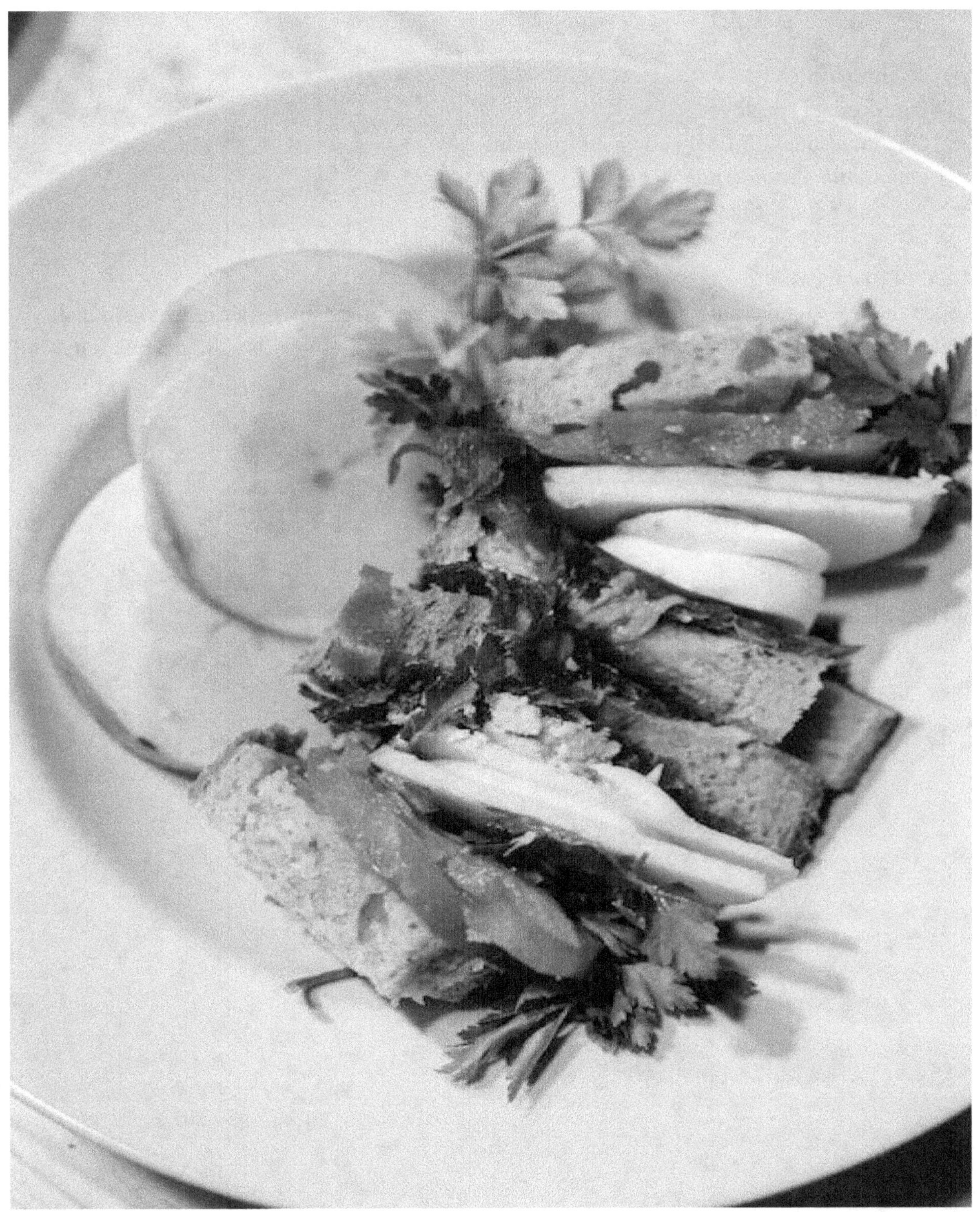

Ingredients:

- 2 tablespoons olive oil
- 4 salmon fillets
- 2 minced garlic cloves
- One tablespoon of finely chopped fresh dill
- One thinly sliced lemon
- Salt and pepper to taste

Method of preparation

1. Adjust the oven temperature to 375°F (190°C) and place parchment paper in a baking dish.
2. Transfer the salmon fillets to the baking dish and dress them with salt, pepper, olive oil, minced garlic, and chopped dill.
3. Place lemon slices on top of each fillet.
4. Bake the salmon for 12 to 15 minutes, or until it is thoroughly done.

Time Required for Preparation: 20 minutes -

Nutritional Value: High in protein, critical vitamins, and omega-3 fatty acids; good for heart health and blood sugar control.

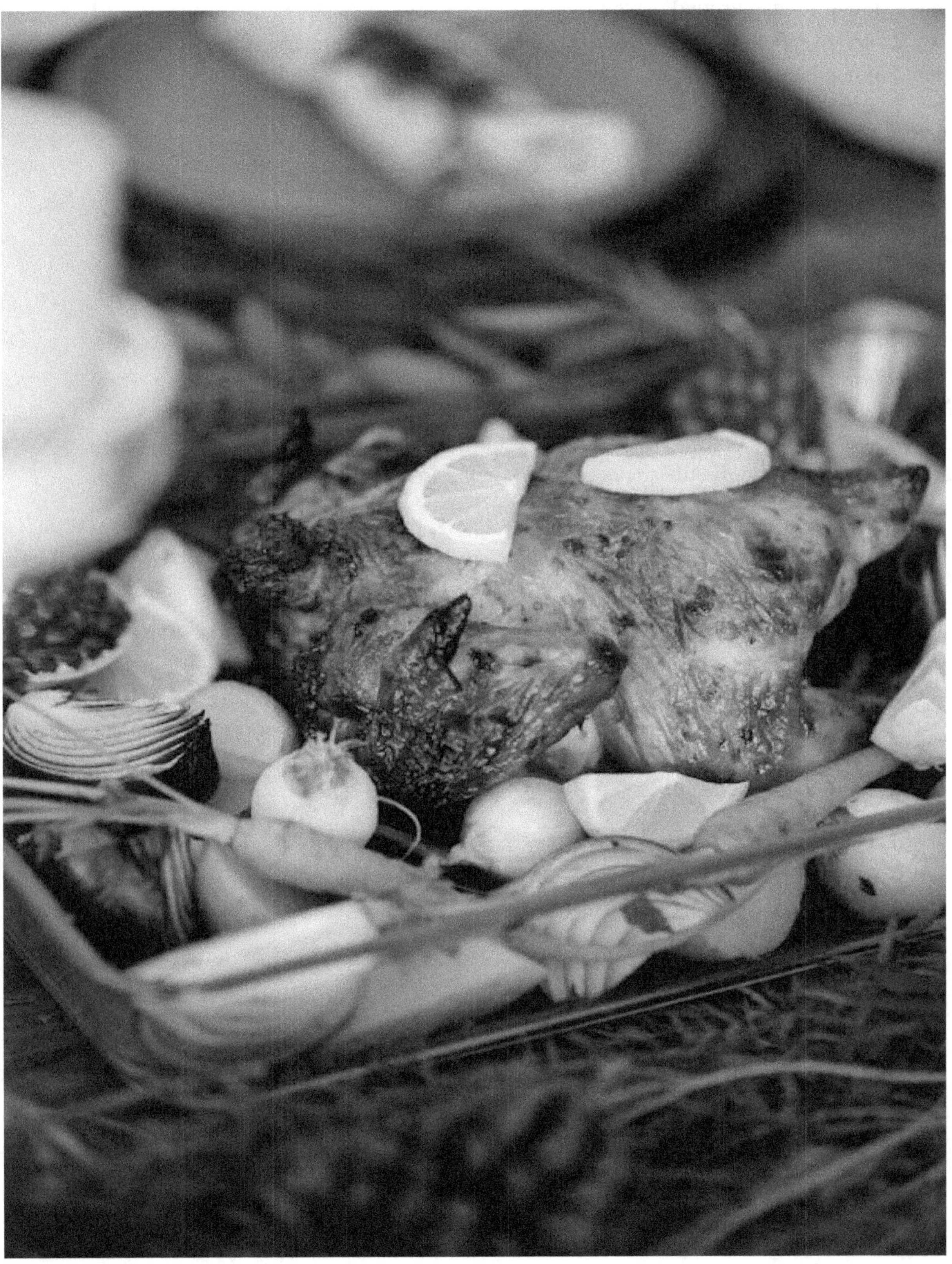

Ingredients:

- 1 pound of lean ground turkey
- 2 cups of mixed vegetables (carrots, broccoli, and bell peppers)
- 2 minced garlic cloves
- Two tablespoons of low-sodium soy sauce
- One tablespoon of sesame oil
- One teaspoon of grated ginger
- To taste, add salt and pepper.

How to prepare:

1. In a large skillet over medium heat, warm the sesame oil.
2. Add the grated ginger and minced garlic, and cook for one minute.
3. Add the turkey meat to the skillet and sear it until it turns brown.
4. Cook the mixed veggies until they are soft, stirring in the soy sauce.

Set Up Time: twenty-five minutes

Nutritional Value: Rich in fiber and lean protein, low in carbohydrates and saturated fat, perfect for controlling blood sugar levels.

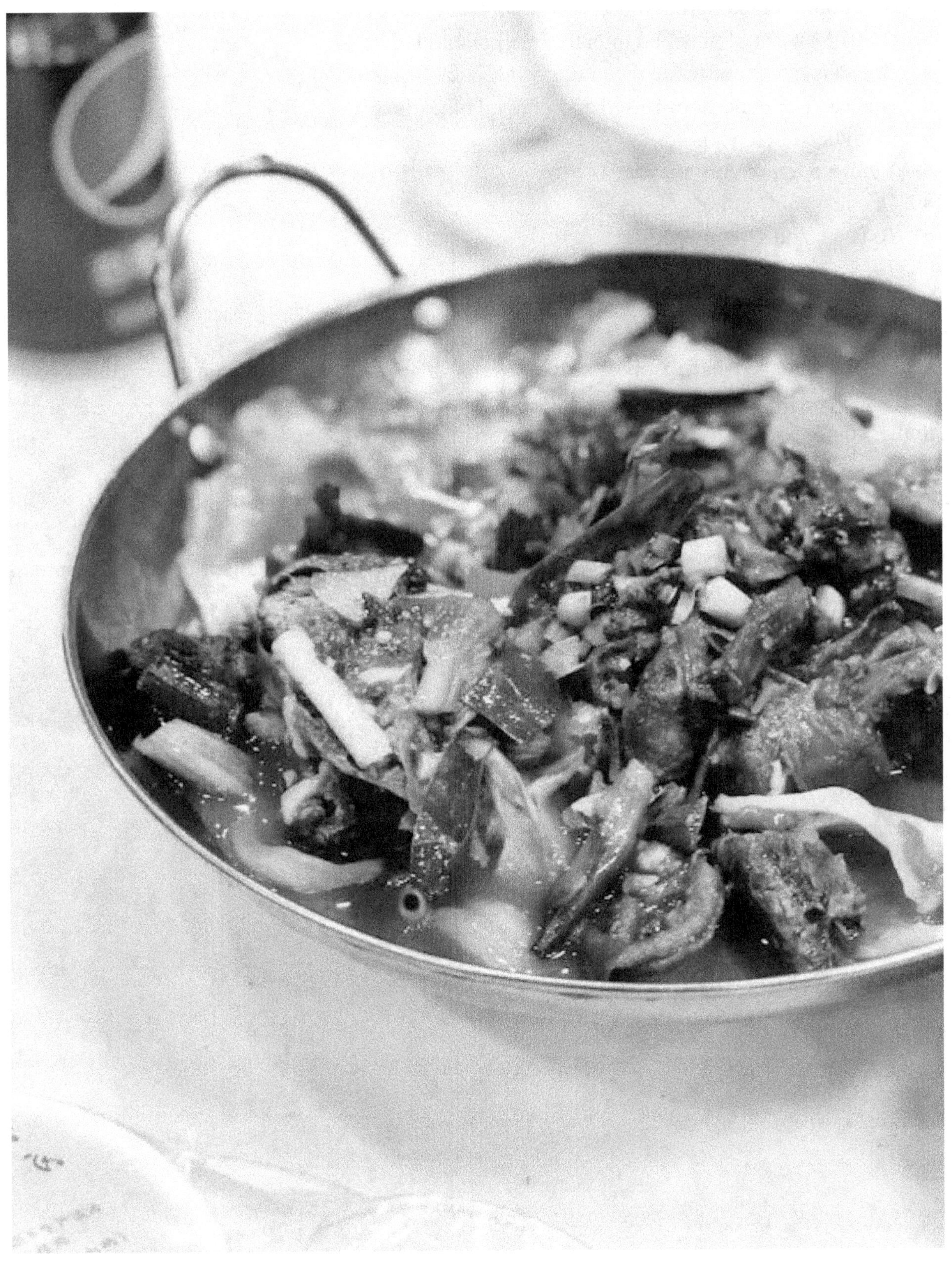

Ingredients:

- One pound of lean ground beef; one chopped onion; two minced garlic cloves
- One 14-oz can of chopped tomatoes without added sugar
- One can (15 oz) of washed and drained kidney beans
- One can (15 ounces) of rinsed and drained black beans
- One sliced bell pepper
- 1 tablespoon of chili powder
- One teaspoon cumin
- To taste, add salt and pepper.

Preparation Method:

1. Brown ground beef, chopped onions, and minced garlic in a big pot.

2. Include the chopped bell pepper, kidney beans, black beans, diced tomatoes, cumin, chili powder, and salt and pepper.

3. Simmer for 20 to 30 minutes over low heat, stirring now and then.

Time Required for Preparation: 40 minutes

Value for Nutrition: Packed with vital nutrients, fiber, and protein, this chili maintains muscular health and gives you steady energy.

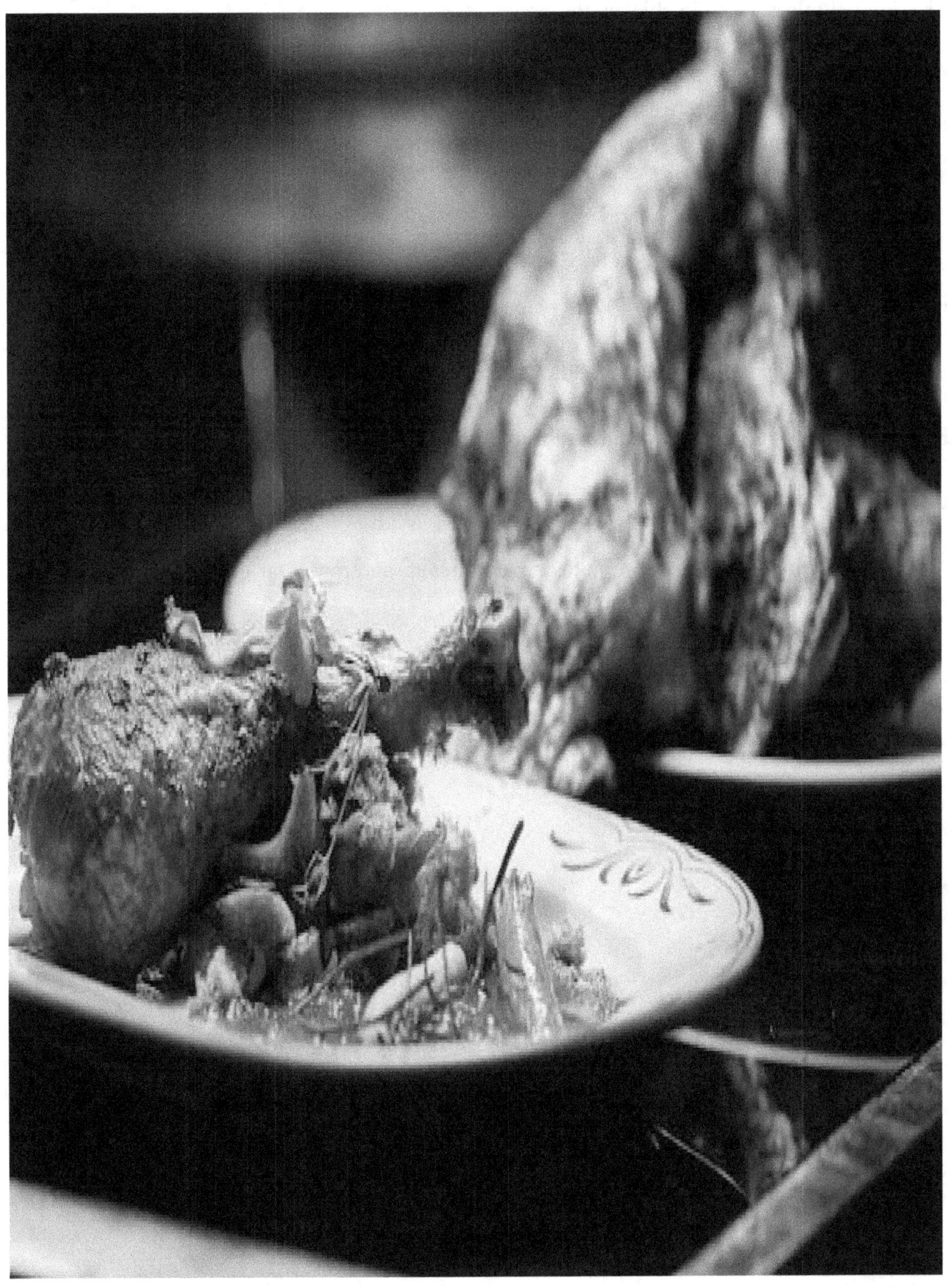

Ingredients:

- Four skinless, bone-in chicken thighs
- Two tablespoons of olive oil
- Two minced garlic cloves
- 1 tablespoon chopped fresh rosemary
- One tablespoon of fresh thyme leaves
- One finely sliced lemon
- To taste, add salt and pepper.

Preparation Method:

1. Preheat the oven to 400°F (200°C) and place parchment paper on a baking pan.

2. Arrange the chicken thighs on the baking sheet and sprinkle with salt, pepper, olive oil, minced garlic, and chopped rosemary and thyme.

3. Lay slices of lemon on top of each thigh.

4. Roast the chicken for 25 to 30 minutes, or until it's well done and has a golden brown color.

Set Up Time: 35 minutes

Value for Nutrition: This dish promotes general health and muscular growth because it is low in added fat and high in protein and micronutrients.

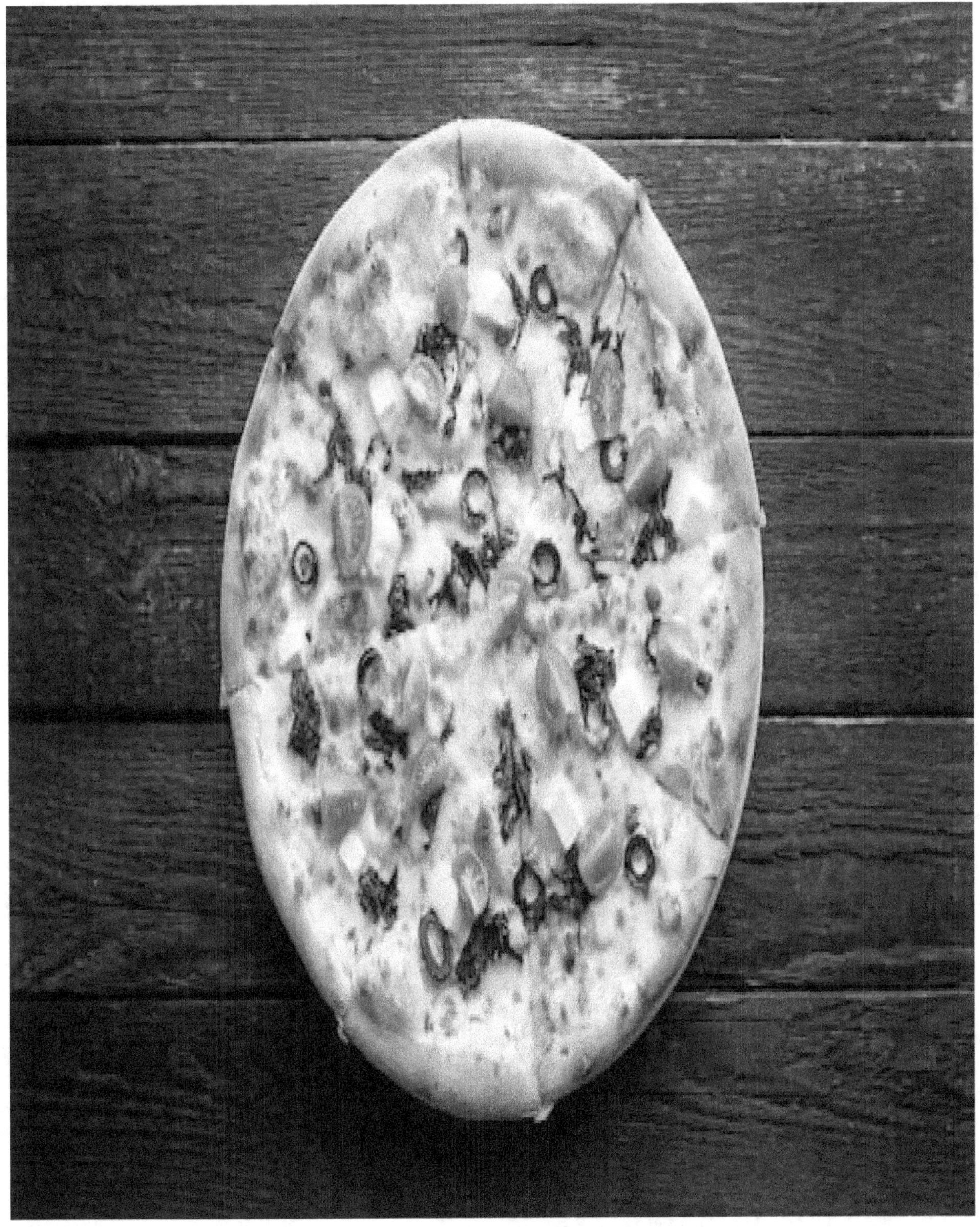

Ingredients:

- 4 fish fillets
- 1 cup chopped cherry tomatoes
- 1/4 cup chopped pitted Kalamata olives
- 2 tablespoons freshly chopped parsley
- One tablespoon of olive oil
- Juiced lemon
- To taste, add salt and pepper.

Method of Preparation:

1. Adjust the oven temperature to 375°F (190°C) and place parchment paper in a baking dish.
2. Transfer the cod fillets to the baking dish and dress them with salt, pepper, lemon juice, and olive oil.
3. Combine chopped parsley, chopped olives, and cherry tomatoes in a basin. Over the fish fillets, spoon the mixture.
4. Bake for 15 to 20 minutes, or until the salmon flakes easily with a fork and is opaque.

Time Required for Preparation: half an hour

Value for Nutrition: This dish, which is rich in antioxidants and omega-3 fatty acids, helps blood sugar regulation and heart health

7. Vegetable and Turkey Kebabs:

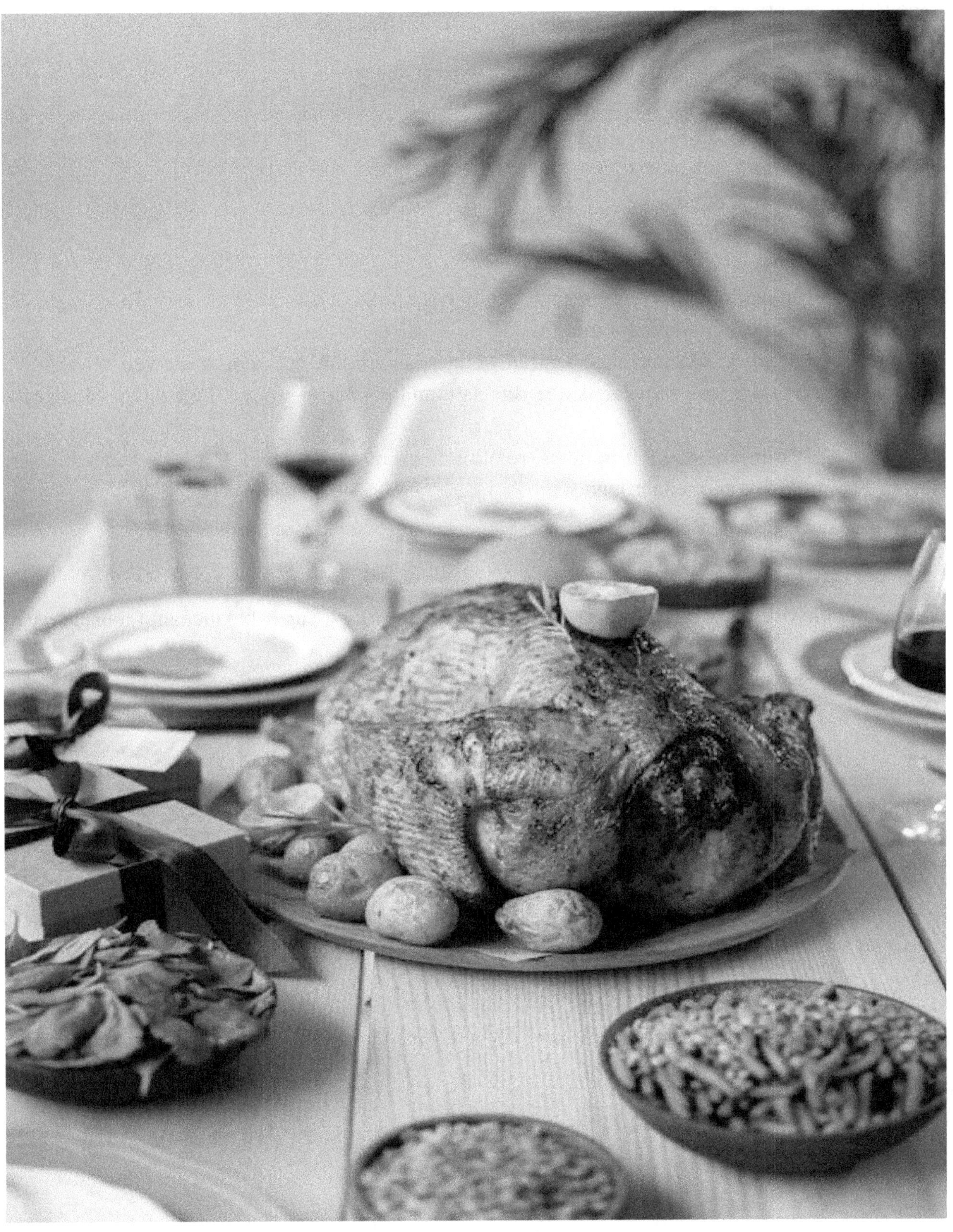

Ingredients:

1-pound turkey breast, cubed

- Two bell peppers, sliced into pieces.
- One slice of zucchini
- One red onion, thinly sliced
- Two tablespoons of olive oil
- minced garlic cloves
- One teaspoon of paprika
- To taste, add salt and pepper.

Method of Preparation:

1. Turn the grill's heat up to medium-high.
2. Thread bell peppers, zucchini slices, onion wedges, and turkey cubes onto skewers.
3. Combine olive oil, paprika, chopped garlic, salt, and pepper in a bowl. Drizzle the blend onto the skewers.
4. Grill the skewers for 8 to 10 minutes, rotating them now and again, until the vegetables are soft and the turkey is cooked through.

Set Up Time:25 minutes

Value for Nutrition: This dish offers vital nutrients for blood sugar balance and muscle repair because it is high in lean protein and low in carbohydrates.

8. Stir-fried beef and broccoli:

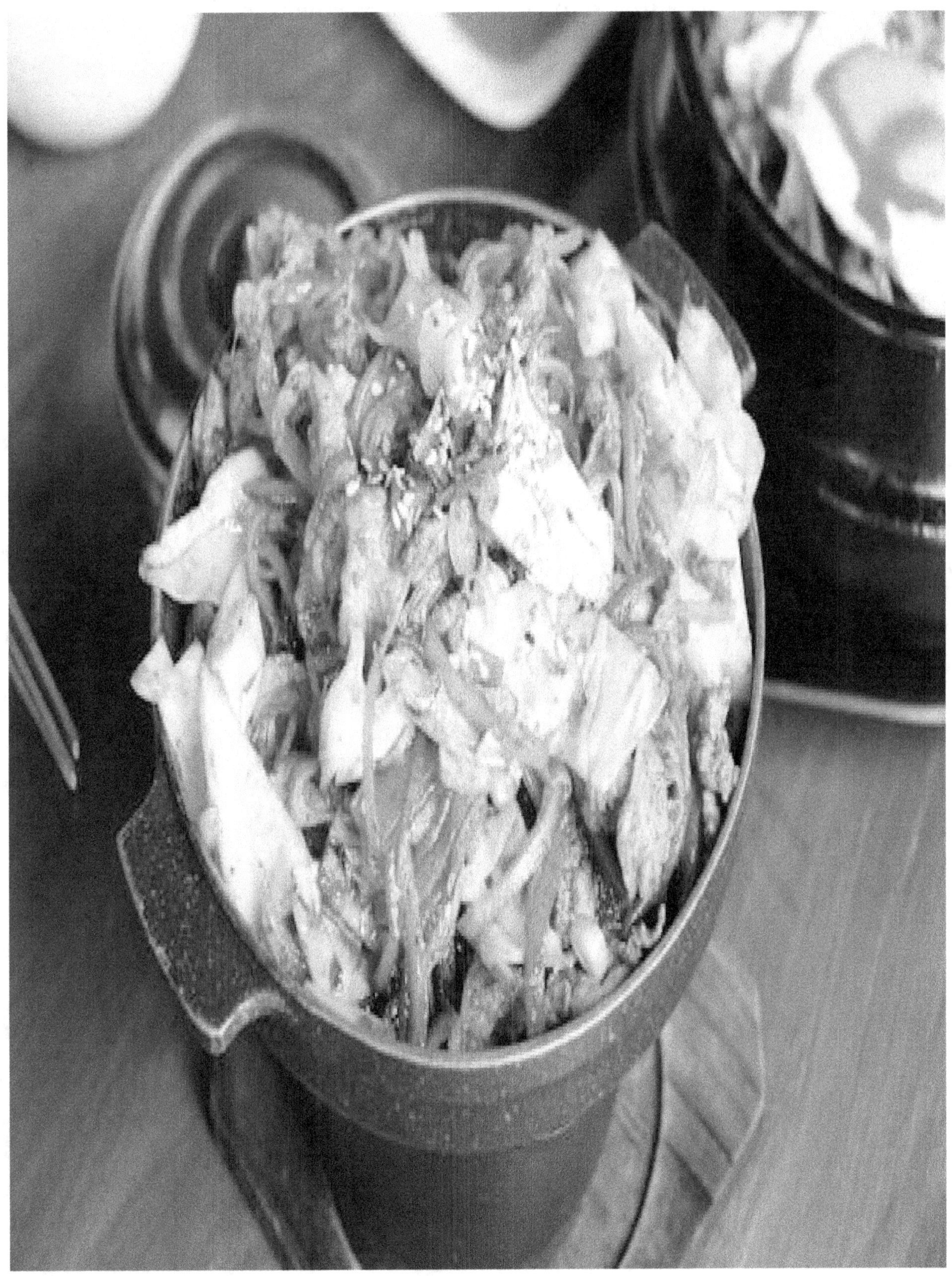

Ingredients:

- One pound of finely cut flank steak and two cups of broccoli florets
- One sliced bell pepper
- Two minced garlic cloves
- 1/4 cup soy sauce with low-sodium
- One tablespoon rice vinegar - One tablespoon sesame oil - One tablespoon cornstarch
- 1 garnish of sesame seeds

How to Prepare:

1. To make the sauce, combine the soy sauce, rice vinegar, sesame oil, and cornstarch in a bowl.
2. Add the flank steak slices and stir-fry them in a skillet over medium-high heat until browned. Take out of the skillet and place aside.
3. Place bell pepper slices, broccoli florets, and minced garlic in the same skillet. Stir-fry the veggies until they become crisp-tender.
4. Place the cooked steak back into the skillet and cover the contents with the sauce. Cook, stirring, for a further two to three minutes.
5. Before serving, garnish with sesame seeds.

Time Required for Preparation: half an hour

Value for Nutrition: For those with diabetes, this stir-fry, which is high in fiber, protein, and vitamins, makes a filling and healthy dinner choice.

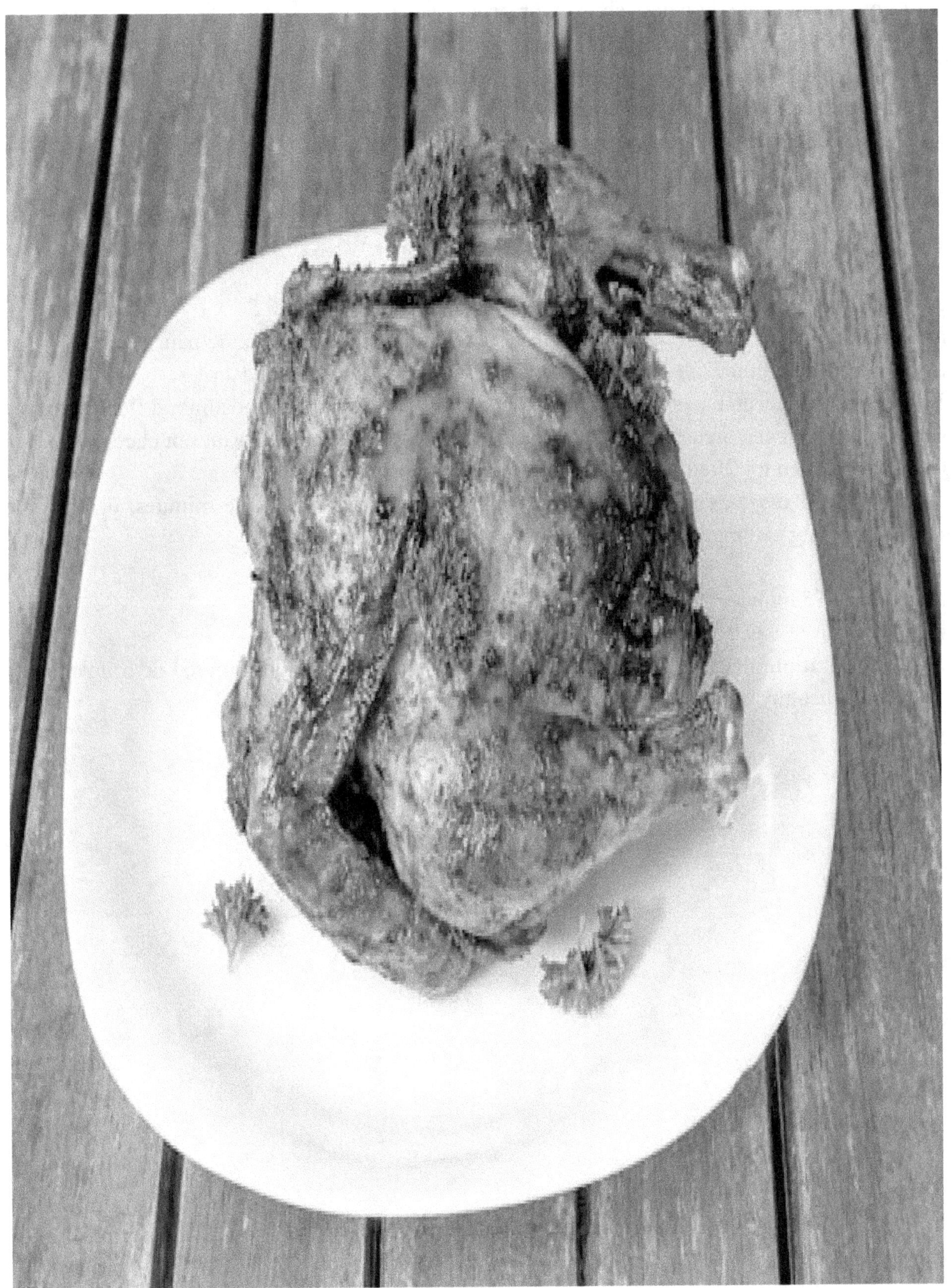

Ingredients:

- Four skinless and boneless chicken breasts
- One cup of sugar-free marinara sauce
- 1/2 cup of mozzarella cheese that has been shredded;
- 1/2 cup of grated Parmesan cheese
- 1 tsp Italian seasoning
- 1/4 cup almond flour
- To taste, add salt and pepper.

Method of Preparation:

1. Preheat the oven to 400°F (200°C) and place parchment paper on a baking pan.
2. Combine almond flour, salt, pepper, and Italian seasoning in a small basin.
3. Transfer each chicken breast to the baking sheet after coating it with the almond flour mixture.
4. Drizzle each chicken breast with marinara sauce and top with grated Parmesan cheese.
5. Bake the chicken for 20 to 25 minutes, or until it is thoroughly done.
6. Add shredded mozzarella cheese on top, then bake for a further five minutes, or until the cheese is bubbling and melted.

Set Up Time: 35 minutes

Value for Nutrition: Rich in calcium and protein, this version of the traditional favorite chicken parmesan is a healthy option that works well for diabetic-friendly meals.

10. Grilled Shrimp with Lemon Garlic:

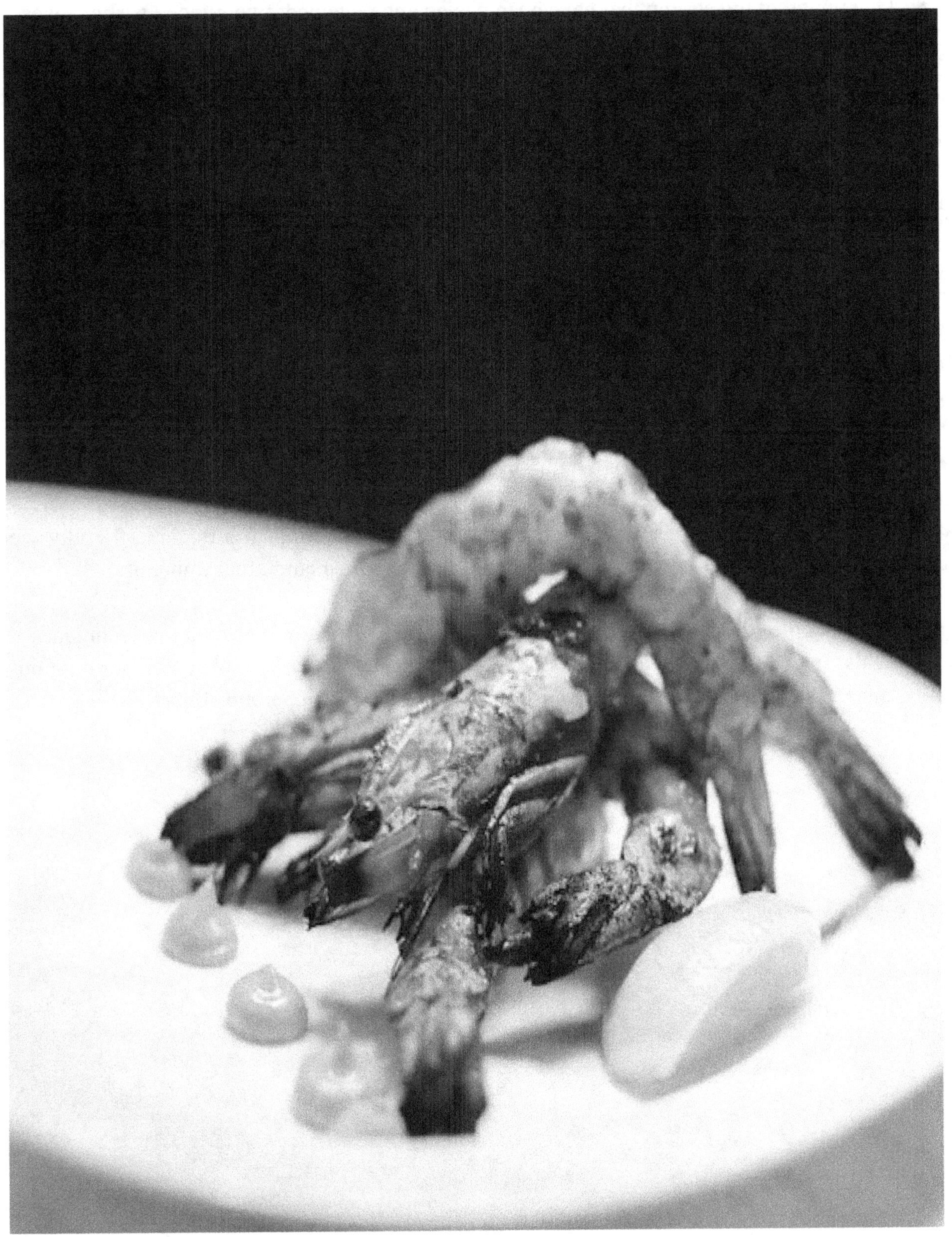

Ingredients:

- One pound of big shrimp that have been peeled and deveined; two minced garlic cloves
- Two tablespoons of olive oil
- One lemon squeezed and sliced
- One teaspoon of smoked paprika
- To taste, add salt and pepper.

How to Prepare:

1. Combine olive oil, smoked paprika, zest and juice of lemons, minced garlic, salt, and pepper in a bowl.
2. Toss the shrimp in the basin to ensure uniform coating. Give the marinade 15 to 20 minutes.
3. Before threading shrimp onto skewers, preheat the grill to medium-high heat.
4. Grill the shrimp skewers for two to three minutes on each side, or until the shrimp turn opaque pink.

Time Required for Preparation: half an hour

Value for Nutrition: This grilled shrimp meal is a tasty addition to a diabetic-friendly diet because it is low in calories and carbohydrates and high in protein and other minerals.

For diabetic people, these meat recipes provide a range of flavors and cooking techniques to make meals interesting and fulfilling. Include them in your meal plan for scrumptious, well-balanced selections that promote blood sugar regulation and general wellness.

CHAPTER 5

FISH AND SEAFOOD RECIPES

Fish and seafood recipes with ingredients, preparation time, method, and nutritional value that are specifically suited for diabetes patients:

1. Grilled Lemon Herb Salmon:

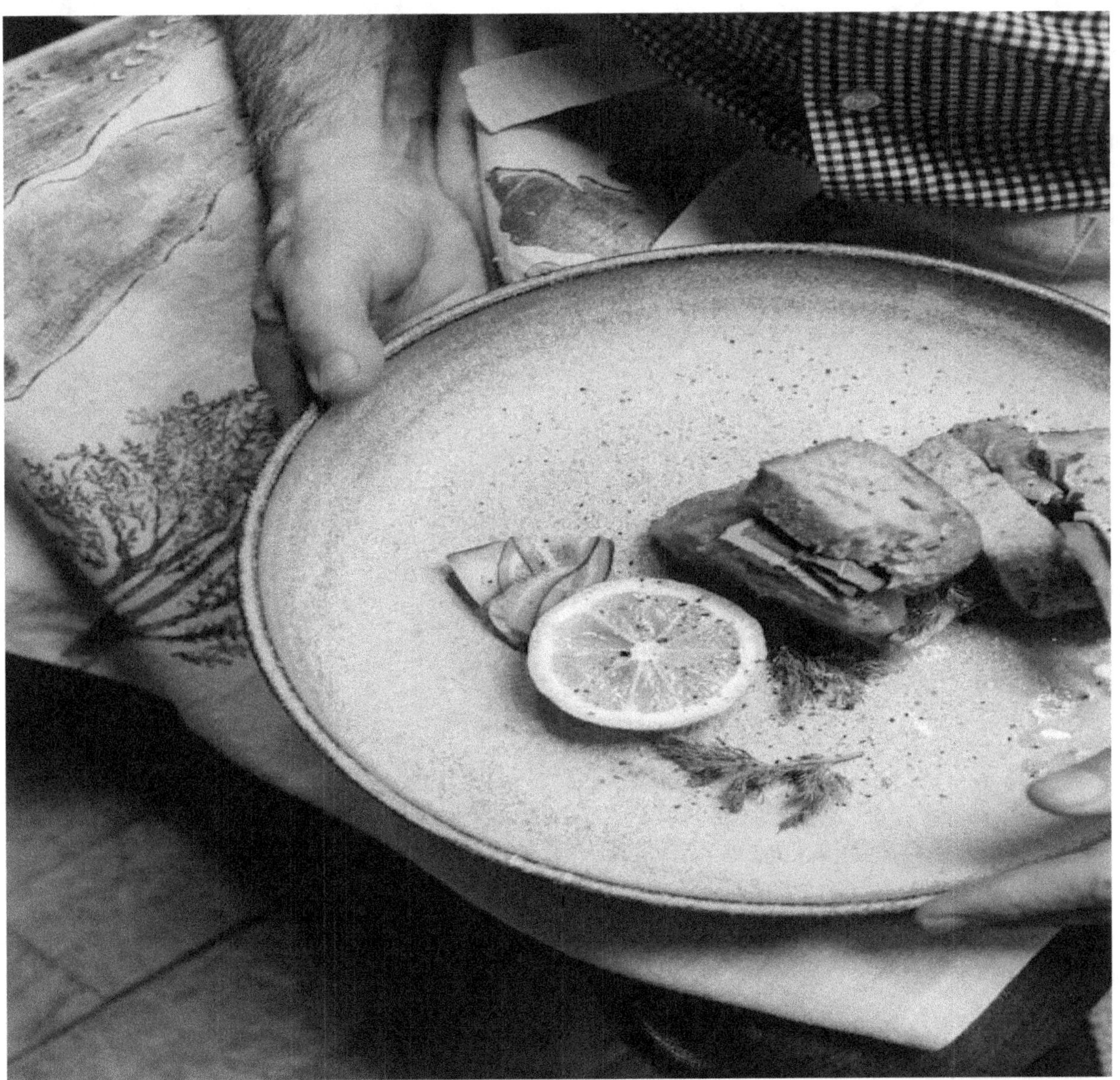

Constitution:

- 2 tablespoons olive oil
- 4 salmon fillets
- 2 minced garlic cloves
- Juiced and zest one lemon;
- One teaspoon of dried dill
- To taste, add salt and pepper.

Preparation Method:

1. Turn the grill's heat to medium.
2. Combine olive oil, salt, pepper, dried dill, lemon zest, lemon juice, and chopped garlic in a bowl.
3. Apply the blend to the salmon fillets.
4. Cook the salmon on the grill for 4–5 minutes on each side, or until it's done.

Time Required for Preparation: 20 minutes

Value for Nutrition: Salmon is high in protein and omega-3 fatty acids, which are vital minerals for blood sugar regulation and heart health.

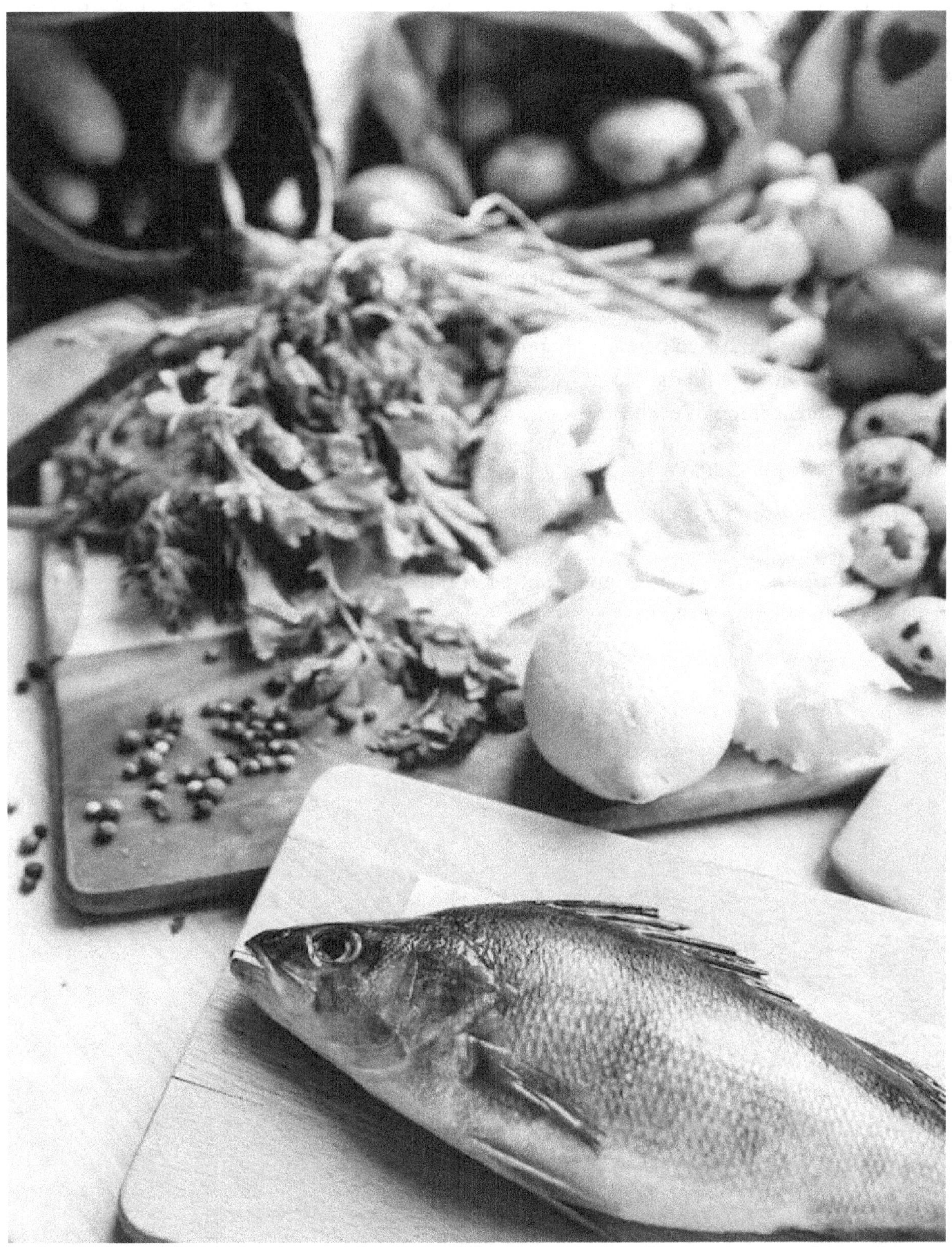

Ingredients:
- 2 tablespoons melted butter
- 4 tilapia fillets
- 2 chopped garlic cloves
- One sliced lemon
- One teaspoon dried parsley
- Adjust with salt and pepper to taste

Method of Preparation:

Preheat the oven to 400°F, or 200°C, and coat a baking dish with oil.

2. Put the fillets of tilapia into the baking dish.

3. Combine melted butter, dried parsley, chopped garlic, salt, and pepper in a small bowl.

4. Cover the tilapia fillets with the butter mixture.

5. Place lemon slices on top of each fillet.

6. Bake the fish for 12 to 15 minutes, or until a fork can easily pierce it.

Time Required for Preparation: 20 minutes

Value for Nutrition: Tilapia is a great option for those with diabetes because it is low in calories and fat and high in protein.

3. Vegetable and Shrimp Stir-Fry:

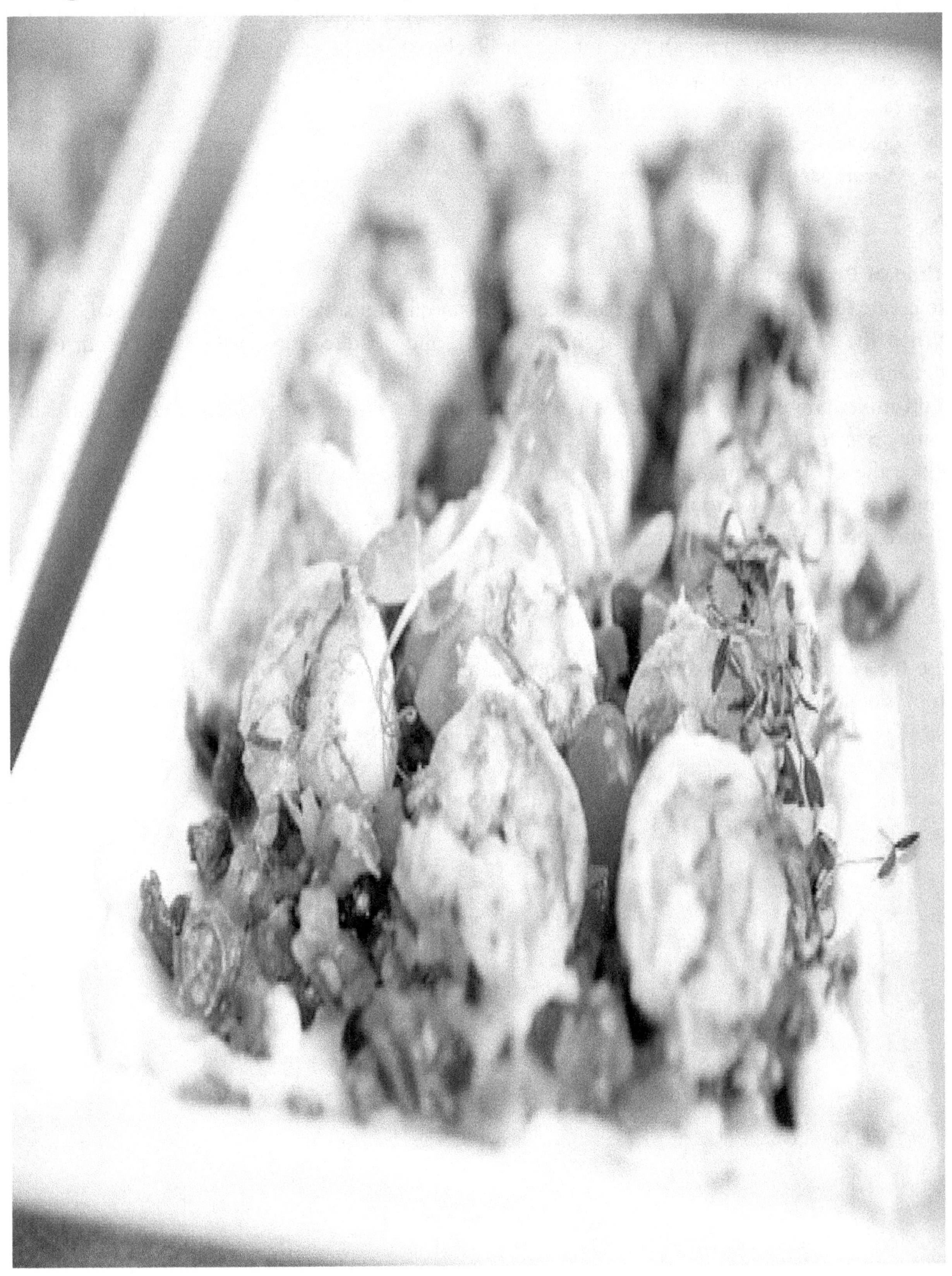

Ingredients:

- One pound of peeled and deveined shrimp; two cups of mixed veggies (broccoli, bell peppers, and snap peas); two minced garlic cloves
- Two tablespoons low-sodium soy sauce
- One tablespoon of sesame oil
- One teaspoon cornstarch
- A garnish of sesame seeds

Method of Preparation:

1. To create the sauce, combine the soy sauce, cornstarch, and sesame oil in a small bowl.

2. When the skillet is hot and the shrimp are pink and opaque, stir-fry them. Take out of the skillet and place aside.

3. Add mixed vegetables and minced garlic to the same skillet. Stir-fry the veggies until they become crisp-tender.

4. Place the cooked shrimp back into the skillet and cover the contents with the sauce. Cook, stirring, for a further two to three minutes.

5. Before serving, garnish with sesame seeds.

Set Up Time: 25 minutes

Value for Nutrition: This shrimp and vegetable stir-fry is low in calories and carbohydrates but high in protein and fiber, making it a great option for diabetic-friendly meals.

4. Grilled Shrimp Skewers with Lemon Garlic:

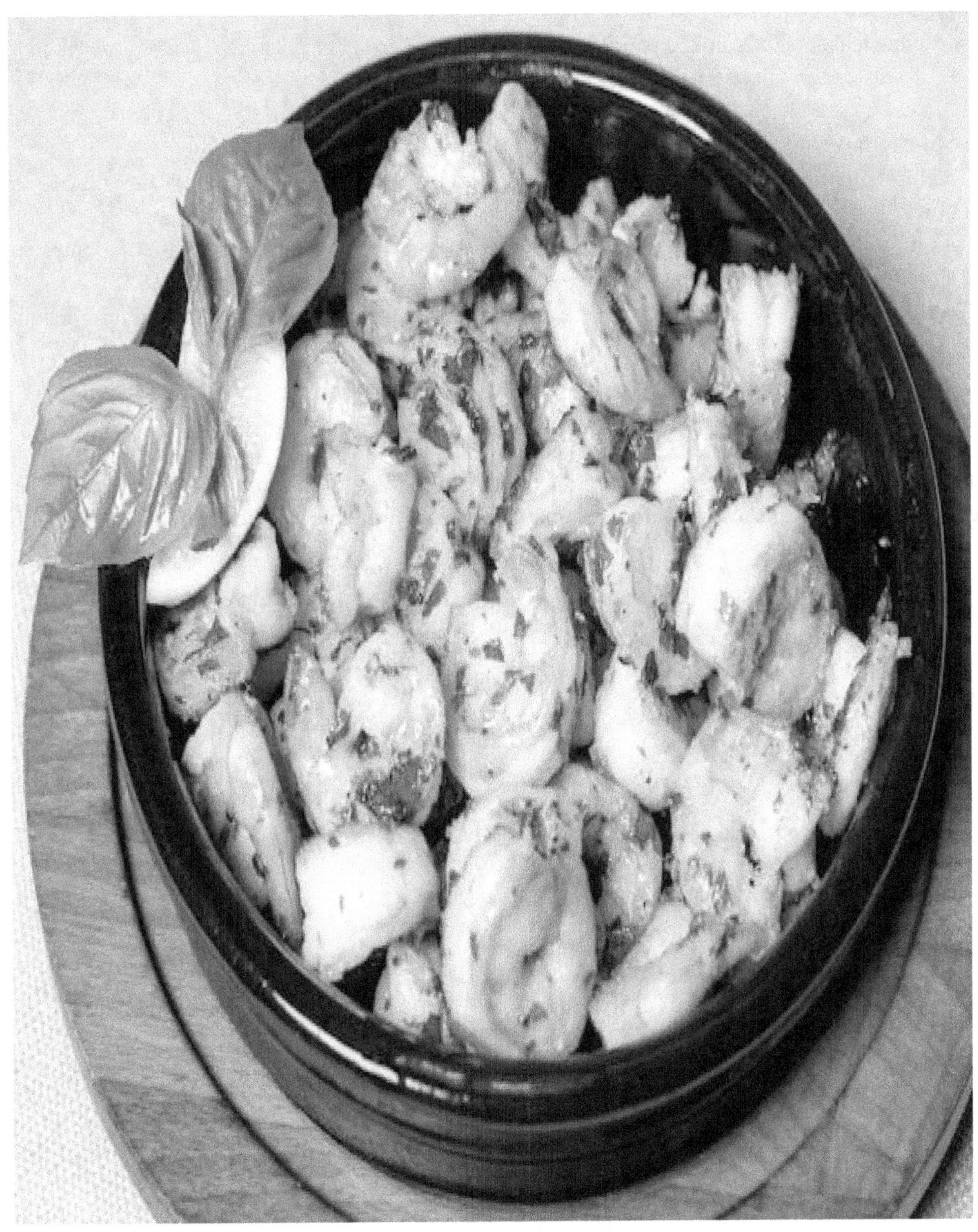

Ingredients:

- One pound of big shrimp that have been peeled and detained; two minced garlic cloves
- Two tablespoons of olive oil
- One lemon squeezed and sliced
- One teaspoon of smoked paprika
- To taste, add salt and pepper.

How to Prepare:

1. Combine olive oil, smoked paprika, zest and juice of lemons, minced garlic, salt, and pepper in a bowl.
2. Toss the shrimp in the basin to ensure uniform coating. Give the marinade 15 to 20 minutes.
3. Before threading shrimp onto skewers, preheat the grill to medium-high heat.
4. Grill the shrimp skewers for two to three minutes on each side, or until the shrimp turn opaque pink.

Time Required for Preparation: half an hour

Value for Nutrition: This grilled shrimp meal is a tasty addition to a diabetic-friendly diet because it is low in calories and carbohydrates and high in protein and other minerals.

5. Garlic Butter Scallops Pan-Seared:

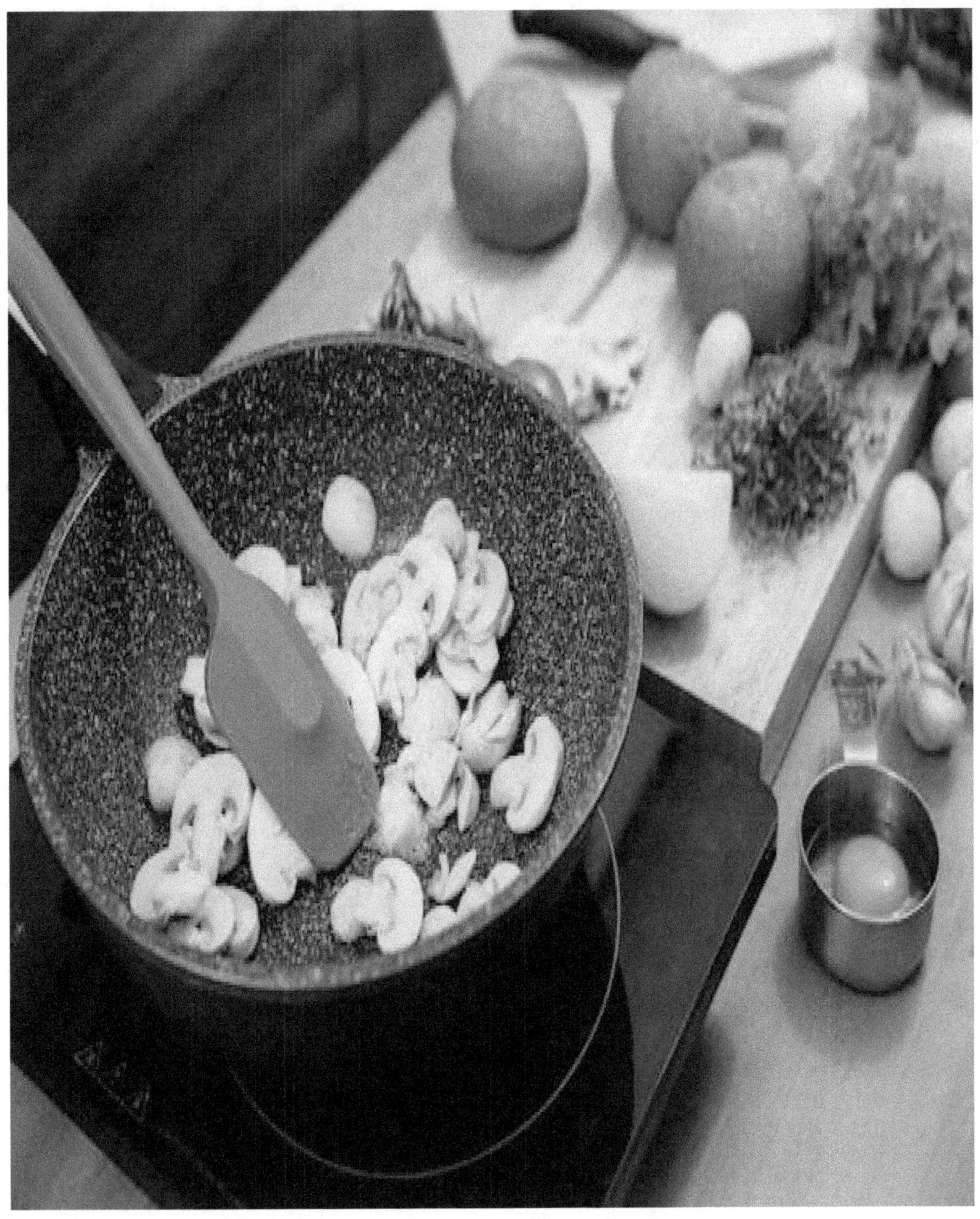

Ingredients:
- One pound of sea scallops; two tablespoons of butter; two chopped garlic cloves
- One tablespoon finely chopped parsley
- To taste, add salt and pepper.

Preparation Method:
1. Use paper towels to pat the scallops dry, then season with salt and pepper.
2. Add butter to a skillet that is heated to medium-high heat.
3. Add the minced garlic to the melted butter and simmer until fragrant.
4. Add the scallops to the skillet and cook them through and golden brown, about two to three minutes per side.
5. Before serving, top the scallops with finely chopped parsley.

Time Required for Preparation: 15 minutes

Value for Nutrition: Because they are low in calories and carbohydrates and a lean protein source, scallops are a good fit for diabetic diets.

Ingredients:
- 2 tablespoons olive oil
- 4 cod fillets
- 2 chopped garlic cloves
- One lemon squeezed and testing
- One tablespoon of freshly chopped dill
- To taste, add salt and pepper.

Preparation Method:
Preheat the oven to 400°F, or 200°C, and coat a baking dish with oil.
2. Fill the baking dish with the cod fillets.
3. Combine olive oil, salt, pepper, chopped dill, lemon zest, lemon juice, and minced garlic in a bowl.
4. Ensure that the fish fillets are evenly coated by pouring the liquid over them.
5. Bake for 15 to 20 minutes, or until a fork can easily pierce the fish.

Set Up Time: twenty-five minutes

Value for Nutrition: Omega-3 fatty acids found in cod, a lean protein source, support heart health and help regulate blood sugar.

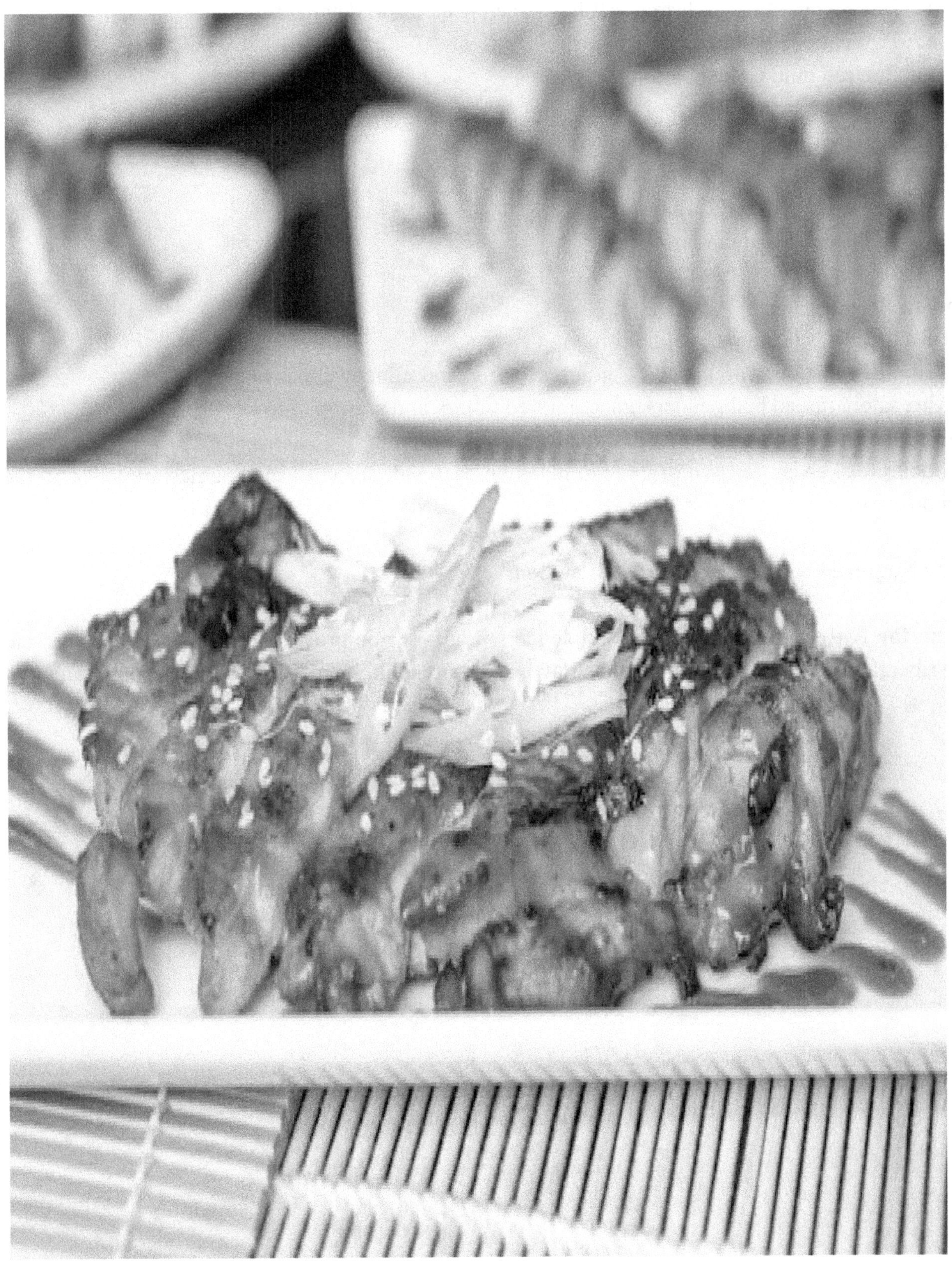

Ingredients:

- One pound of large shrimp that have been peeled and detained
- Two chunky bell peppers
- One red onion, sliced into pieces
- One slice of zucchini
- Two tablespoons of olive oil
- Two minced garlic cloves
- One tablespoon of Cajun spice
- To taste, add salt and pepper.

How to Prepare:

1. Turn the grill's heat up to medium-high.
2. Combine olive oil, salt, pepper, Cajun seasoning, and minced garlic in a basin.
3. Alternately thread bell peppers, zucchini, red onion, and shrimp onto skewers.
4. Give the skewers a light coating of the Cajun spice mixture.
5. Cook the skewers for two to three minutes on each side, or until the veggies are soft and the shrimp are pink.

Time Required for Preparation: Half an hour

Value for Nutrition: The shrimp and veggies in this recipe provide a good amount of protein and fiber, and the Cajun seasoning adds flavor without adding extra calories or carbohydrates.

Ingredients:

- Four fillets of tilapia
- 1/4 cup of finely grated Parmesan cheese
- 2 tablespoons of mayonnaise
- 1-tablespoon lemon juice
- 1/2 tsp. powdered garlic
- A half-tsp of dried basil
- To taste, add salt and pepper.

Preparation Method:

1. Preheat the oven to 400°F (200°C) and place parchment paper on a baking pan.
2. Combine grated Parmesan cheese, dried basil, lemon juice, mayonnaise, garlic powder, and salt & pepper in a bowl.
3. Put the tilapia fillets on the ready baking sheet.
4. Evenly cover each fillet's top with the Parmesan mixture.
5. Bake for 12 to 15 minutes, or until the topping is golden brown and the fish flakes readily with a fork.

Time Required for Preparation: 20 minutes

Nutritional Value: The Parmesan crust adds taste without substantially raising the carb count, and the tilapia provide protein, making it appropriate for diabetic diets.

Ingredients:
- 2 tablespoons olive oil
- 4 swordfish steaks
- 2 minced garlic cloves
- One lemon squeezed and sliced
- One teaspoon dried oregano
- Adjust with salt and pepper to taste.

Method of Preparation:
1. Grease a baking dish and preheat the broiler.
2. Put the swordfish steaks in the ready baking dish.
3. Combine olive oil, dried oregano, lemon zest, lemon juice, minced garlic, salt, and pepper in a bowl.
4. Apply the mixture on the steaks of swordfish.
5. Fish should be opaque and flake readily with a fork after 6 to 8 minutes under the broiler.

Time Required for Preparation: 20 minutes

Value for Nutrition: Omega-3 fatty acids and protein found in swordfish can help regulate blood sugar and strengthen heart function.

Ingredients:
- Four mahi mahi fillets and two tablespoons of Cajun seasoning
- 1 lemon, sliced into wedges
- 2 tablespoons olive oil
- Salt according to taste

Method of Preparation:
1. Evenly coat the mahi mahi fillets on both sides with salt and Cajun seasoning.
2. In a skillet over medium-high heat, warm the olive oil.
3. When the skillet is heated, add the mahi mahi fillets and cook for 4–5 minutes on each side, or until the fish is opaque and flake readily.
4. Accompany the fish with lemon slices so that it can be squeezed.

Time Needed for Preparation: 15 minutes

Value for Nutrition: Mahi is appropriate for diabetic diets since it is a lean source of protein, full of vital minerals, and does not affect blood sugar levels.

These recipes for fish and seafood take into account the nutritional needs of people with diabetes while providing a range of tastes and nutrients. They support diabetics' general health and well-being by offering protein, good fats, and vital vitamins and minerals without raising blood sugar levels.

CHAPTER 6

SOUP RECIPES

Diabetic patients might benefit from these soup recipes, which include information on ingredients, preparation time, method, and nutritional content.

1. Lentil and Vegetable Soup:

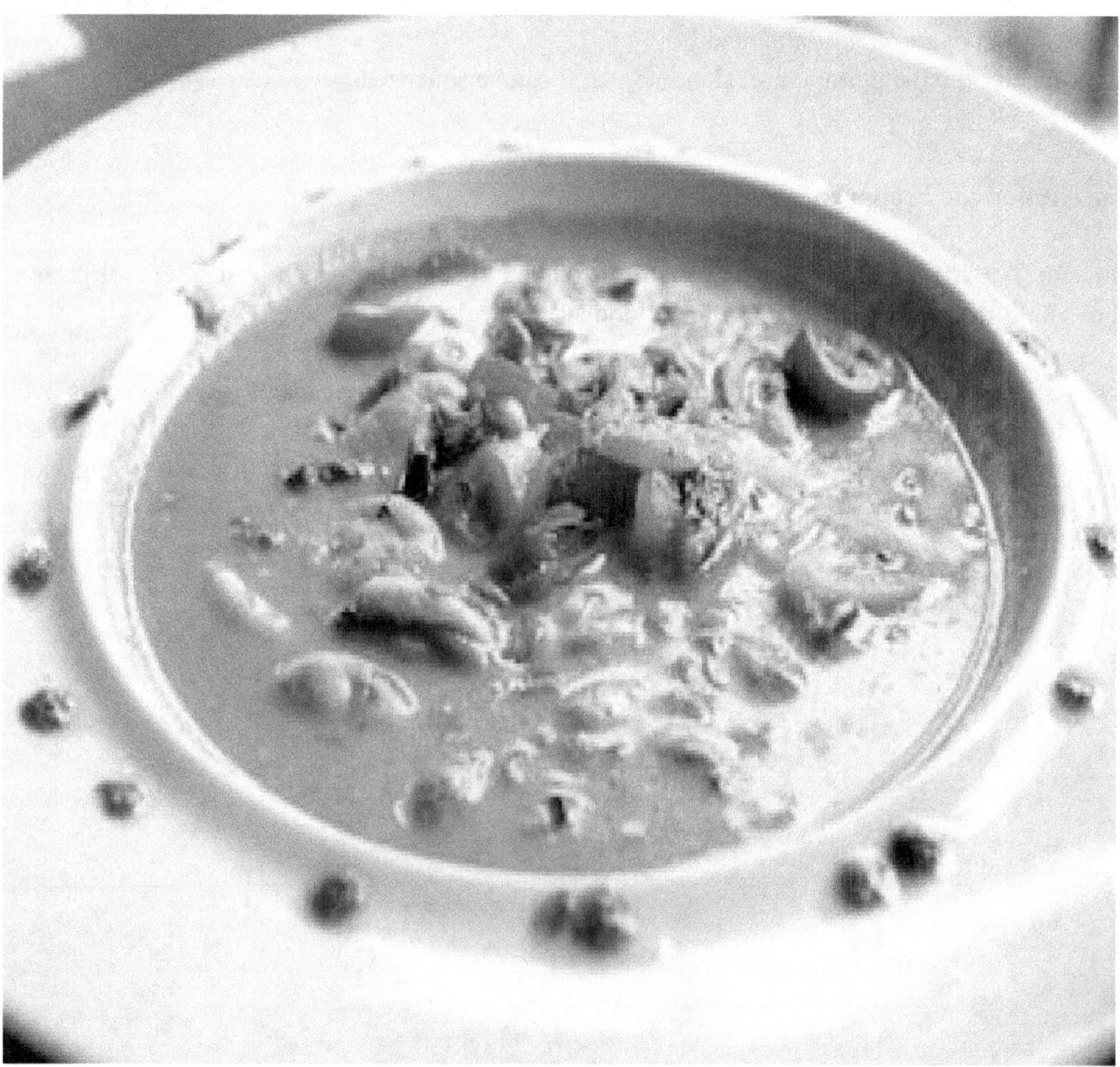

Ingredients:

- One cup of lentils; two sliced carrots; two diced celery stalks; one diced onion
- Three minced garlic cloves
- Six cups vegetable broth
- One teaspoon cumin
- One teaspoon paprika
- To taste, add salt and pepper.

How to Prepare:

1. Saute chopped celery, carrots, onions, and garlic in a big pot until they become tender.
2. Include the lentils, paprika, cumin, vegetable broth, salt, and pepper. Heat till boiling.
3. Once the lentils are soft, reduce the heat and simmer for 20 to 25 minutes.
4. Present warm.

Time Required for Preparation: forty minutes

Value for Nutrition: This soup, which is low in calories and high in fiber, is also a wonderful source of protein, vitamins, and minerals, all of which help to maintain stable blood sugar level.

2. Vegetable and Chicken Soup:

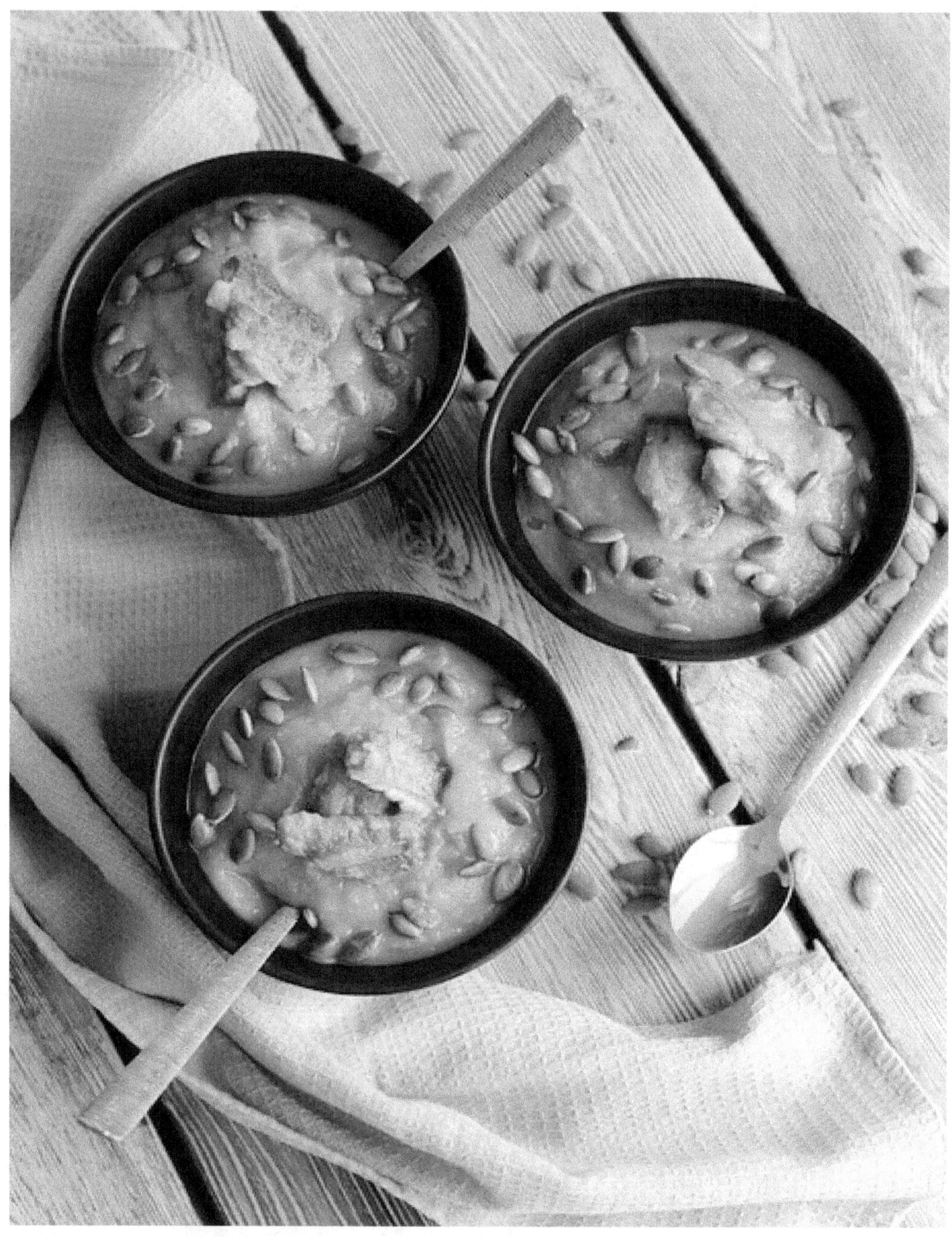

Ingredients:

- One pound of chopped, skinless, boneless chicken breast;
- Four cups of low-sodium chicken broth;
- Two sliced carrots
- 2 sliced celery stalks
- 1 diced onion
- 2 minced garlic cloves
- One teaspoon of dried thyme
- To taste, add salt and pepper.

Preparation Method:

1. Cook the diced chicken in a big pot until it's no longer pink. Take out and place aside.

2. Saute chopped celery, carrots, onions, and garlic in the same pot until they become tender.

Put the cooked chicken back into the pot. Add the dried thyme and chicken broth. Heat till boiling.

4. Once the vegetables are soft, reduce the heat and simmer for 20 to 25 minutes.

5. Before serving, add salt and pepper to taste.

Set Up Time: thirty-five minutes

Value for Nutrition: This soup is low in calories and carbohydrates and high in protein and vitamins, making it a good choice for people with diabetes.

3. White Bean and Spinach Soup:

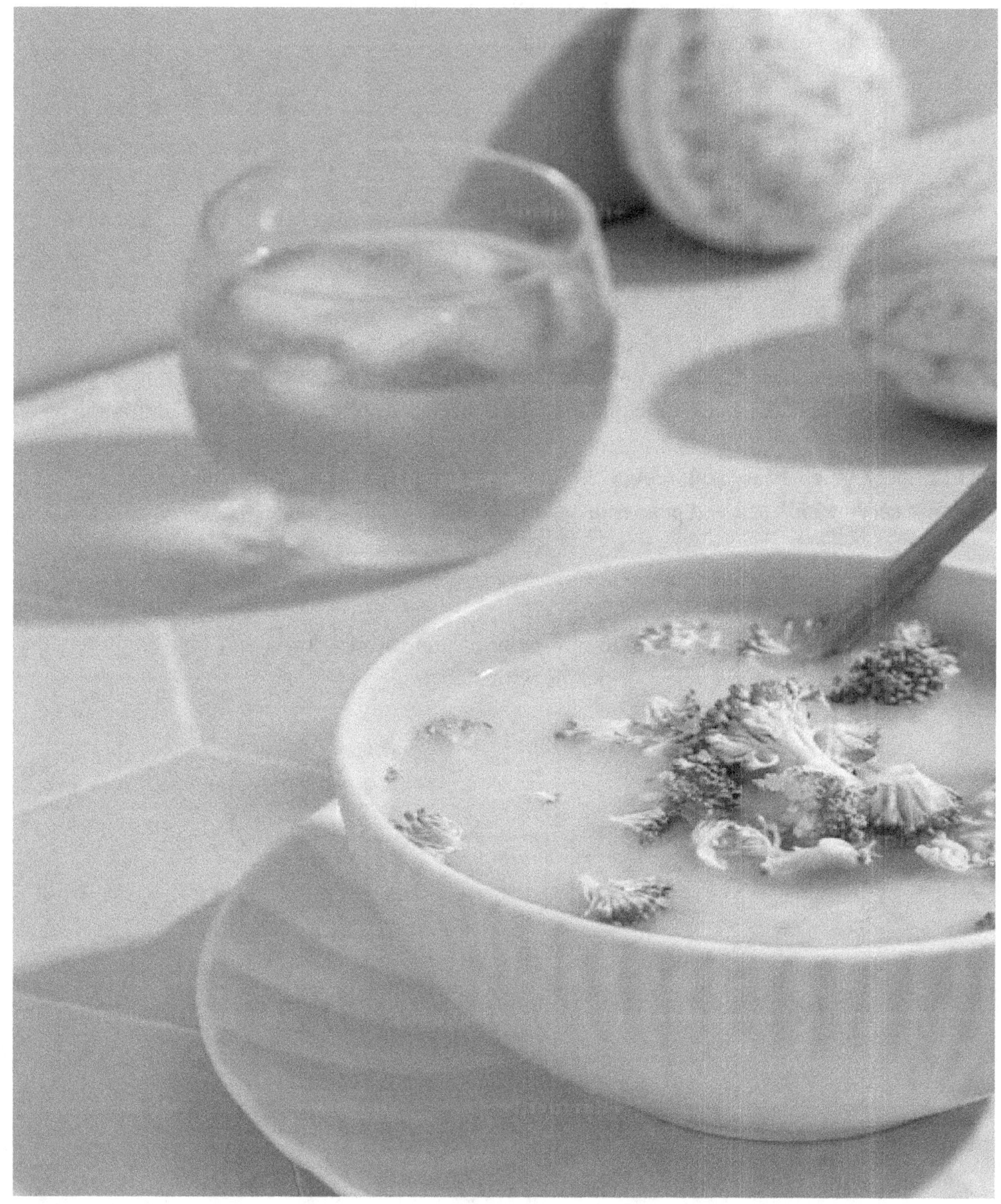

Ingredients:

- 2 tablespoons olive oil
- 1 chopped onion
- 3 minced garlic cloves
- 4 cups of vegetable broth
- 2 cans (15 oz each) of washed and drained white beans
- Four cups of raw spinach
- One teaspoon of dried thyme
- To taste, add salt and pepper.

How to Prepare:

1. Heat the olive oil in a big pot over medium heat. Diced onions and garlic should be sautéed until tender.

2. Include the dried thyme, white beans, and vegetable broth. Heat through to a simmer.

3. To thicken the soup while retaining some whole beans, partially mix the soup using an immersion blender.

4. Add the fresh spinach leaves and boil until the spinach wilts, about 5 more minutes.

5. Before serving, add salt and pepper for seasoning.

Time Required for Preparation: half an hour

Value for Nutrition: This soup, which is low in calories and carbohydrates and rich in iron, protein, and fiber from white beans and spinach, is a great choice for diabetic diets.

4. Sweet Basil Tomato Soup:

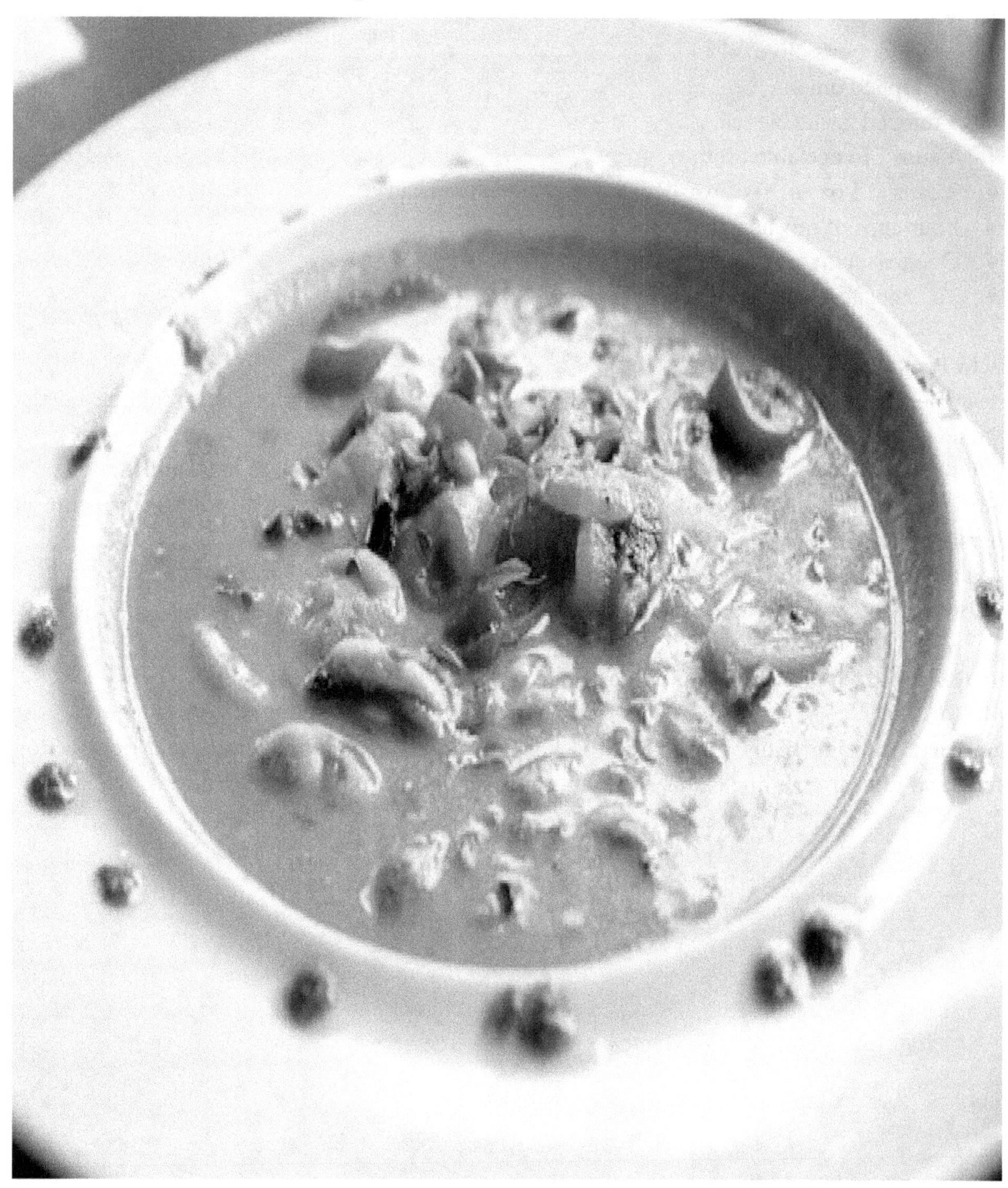

Components:

- 2 tablespoons olive oil
- 1 chopped onion
- 3 minced garlic cloves
- Two 28-ounce cans each Crushed tomatoes
- 4 cups vegetable broth low in sodium
- 1/4 cup freshly chopped basil
- To taste, add salt and pepper.

Method of Preparation:

1. Heat the olive oil in a big pot over medium heat. Diced onions and garlic should be sautéed until tender.
2. Include the veggie broth and smashed tomatoes. Heat through to a simmer.
3. To allow the flavors to mingle, simmer for 15 to 20 minutes.
4. Before serving, add the freshly cut basil and season with salt and pepper.

Set Up Time: Twenty-five Minutes

Nutritional Value: This soup is a good choice for people with diabetes because it is low in calories and carbohydrates and high in vitamins and antioxidants.

5. Soup with Broccoli and Cheddar:

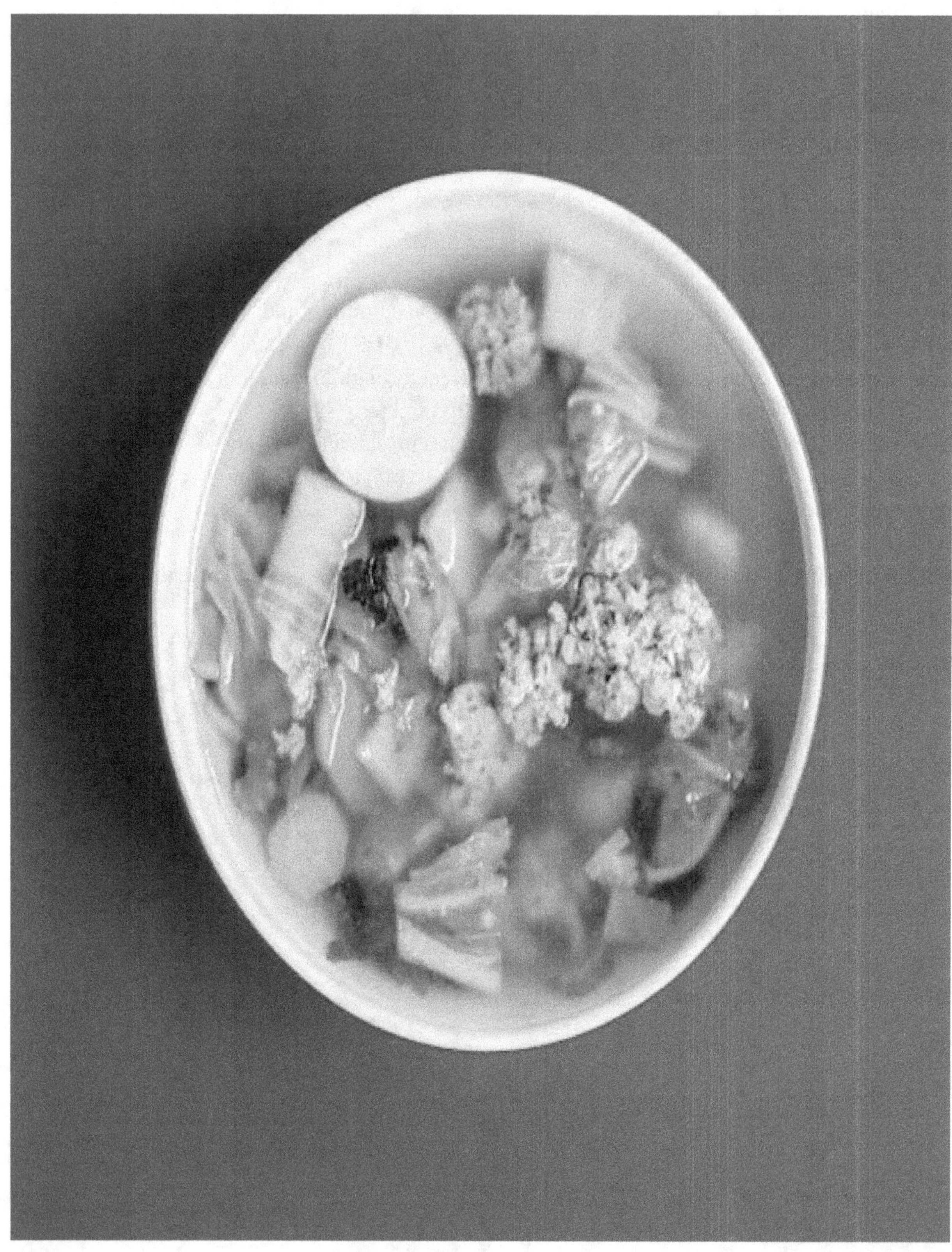

Ingredients:

- 2 tablespoons butter
- 1 chopped onion
- 3 minced garlic cloves
- 4 cups chopped broccoli florets
- 4 cups low-sodium vegetable broth
- One cup of shredded cheddar cheese
- One cup of milk (you can use unsweetened almond milk if you're lactose intolerant).
- To taste, add salt and pepper.

Preparation Method:

1. Melt butter in a big pot over medium heat. Diced onions and garlic should be sautéed until tender.
2. Include chopped broccoli florets and vegetable broth. Heat till boiling.
3. Simmer the broccoli for 15 to 20 minutes over low heat, or until it is soft.
4. Puree the soup with an immersion blender until it's smooth.
5. Add the milk and shredded cheddar cheese, stirring until the cheese melts and the soup is well cooked.
6. Before serving, add salt and pepper for seasoning.

Time Required for Preparation: Half an hour

Value for Nutrition: If portions are monitored, this soup's moderate calorie and carb content, along with its protein, calcium, and fiber content, make it a good choice for diabetic diets.

6. Cookery Soup with Mexican Chicken:

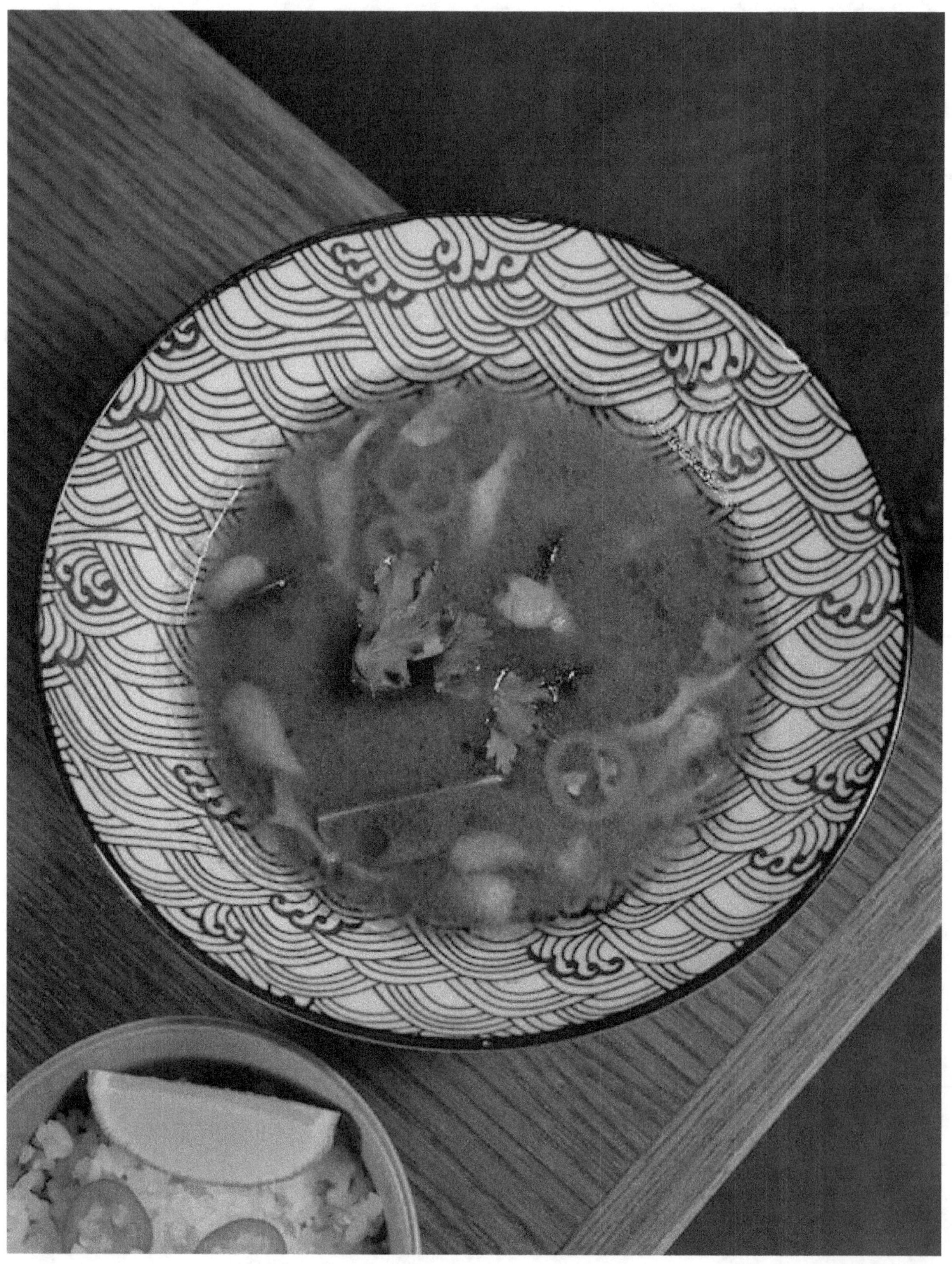

Containments:

- 1 pound of diced, skinless, boneless chicken breast
- 4 cups low-sodium chicken broth
- 1 can (15 oz) of diced tomatoes
- 1 diced bell pepper
- 1 chopped onion
- 2 minced garlic cloves
- A tsp of chili powder
- One teaspoon of ground cumin
- Season with salt and pepper
- Finely slice fresh cilantro (to garnish)

How to Prepare:

1. Cook the diced chicken in a big pot until it's no longer pink. Take out and place aside.
2. Saute the diced onions, bell pepper, and garlic in the same pot until they become tender.
3. Include the diced tomatoes, chicken stock, ground cumin, chili powder, salt, and pepper. Heat till boiling.
4. Simmer for 15 to 20 minutes on low heat.
5. Add the cooked chicken to the pot and let it boil for a further five minutes.
6. Before serving, garnish with finely chopped fresh cilantro.

Time Required for Preparation: 35 minutes

Nutritional Worth: This soup is low in calories and carbohydrates and high in protein and fiber, making it a good choice for people with diabetes.

7. Vegetable and Turkey Soup:

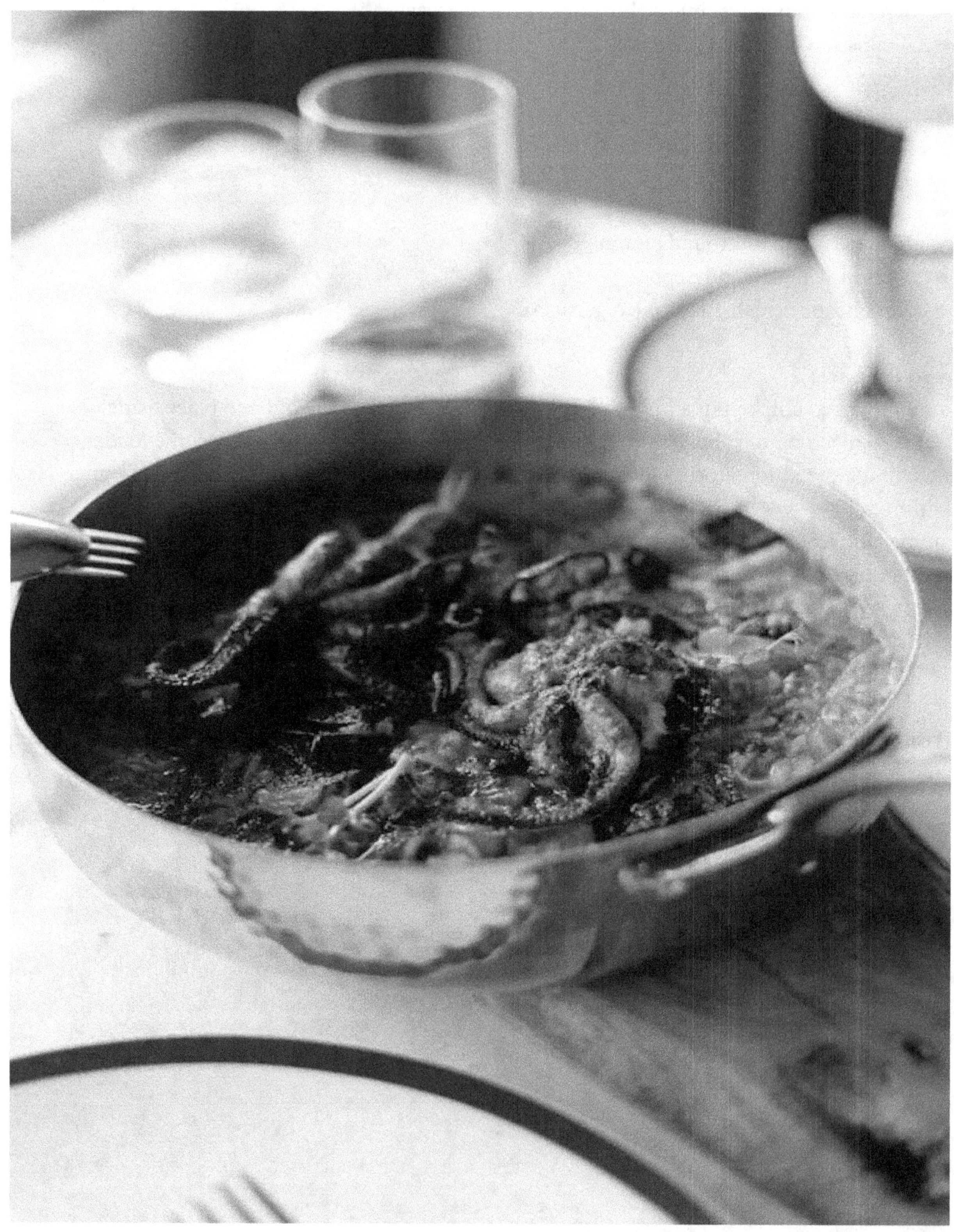

Ingredients:

- One pound of ground turkey; four cups of low-sodium chicken broth; two chopped carrots; two diced celery stalks; one diced onion; and two minced garlic cloves
- One teaspoon of dried thyme
- To taste, add salt and pepper.

Method of Preparation:

1. Brown the ground turkey in a large pot. Eliminate surplus fat and reserve.
2. Saute chopped celery, carrots, onions, and garlic in the same pot until they become tender.
3. Return the cooked ground turkey to the saucepan. Add the dried thyme and chicken broth. Heat till boiling.
4. Once the vegetables are soft, reduce the heat and simmer for 20 to 25 minutes.
5. Before serving, add salt and pepper for seasoning.

Time Required for Preparation: forty minutes

Value for Nutrition: This soup has a low influence on blood sugar levels and is high in lean protein from the turkey as well as important vitamins and minerals.

8. Soup de Minestra:

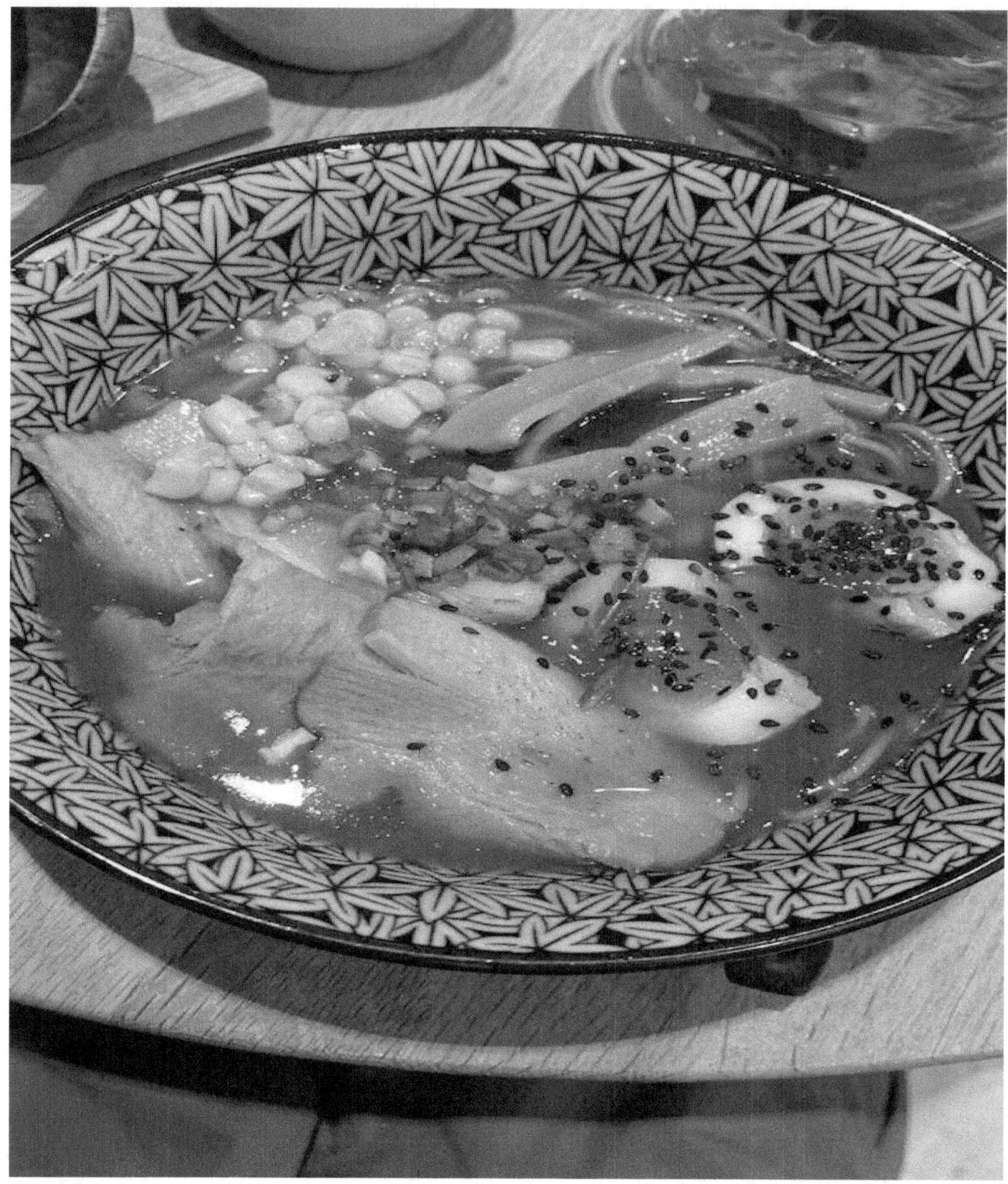

Components:

- 2 tablespoons olive oil
- 1 chopped onion
- 2 diced carrots
- Two chopped celery stalks
- Three minced garlic cloves
- Four cups of low-sodium vegetable broth; one can (15 oz) chopped tomatoes; and one can (15 oz) kidney beans, drained and rinsed
- Chopped green beans, one cup
- 1/2 cup of little pasta, such dialing or macaroni
- One teaspoon dried oregano
- To taste, add salt and pepper.

How to Prepare:

1. Heat the olive oil in a big pot over medium heat. Diced celery, carrots, onions, and garlic should be sautéed until tender.

2. Include the pasta, kidney and green beans, dry oregano, chopped tomatoes, vegetable broth, and salt and pepper. Heat till boiling.

3. After the pasta is cooked and the vegetables are soft, reduce the heat and simmer for 20 to 25 minutes.

4. Present warm.

Time Required for Preparation: 45 minutes

Value for Nutrition: This soup is a healthy option for those with diabetes since it is full of fiber, protein, and vitamins from the vegetables and beans.

9. Thai Coconut Curry Soup:

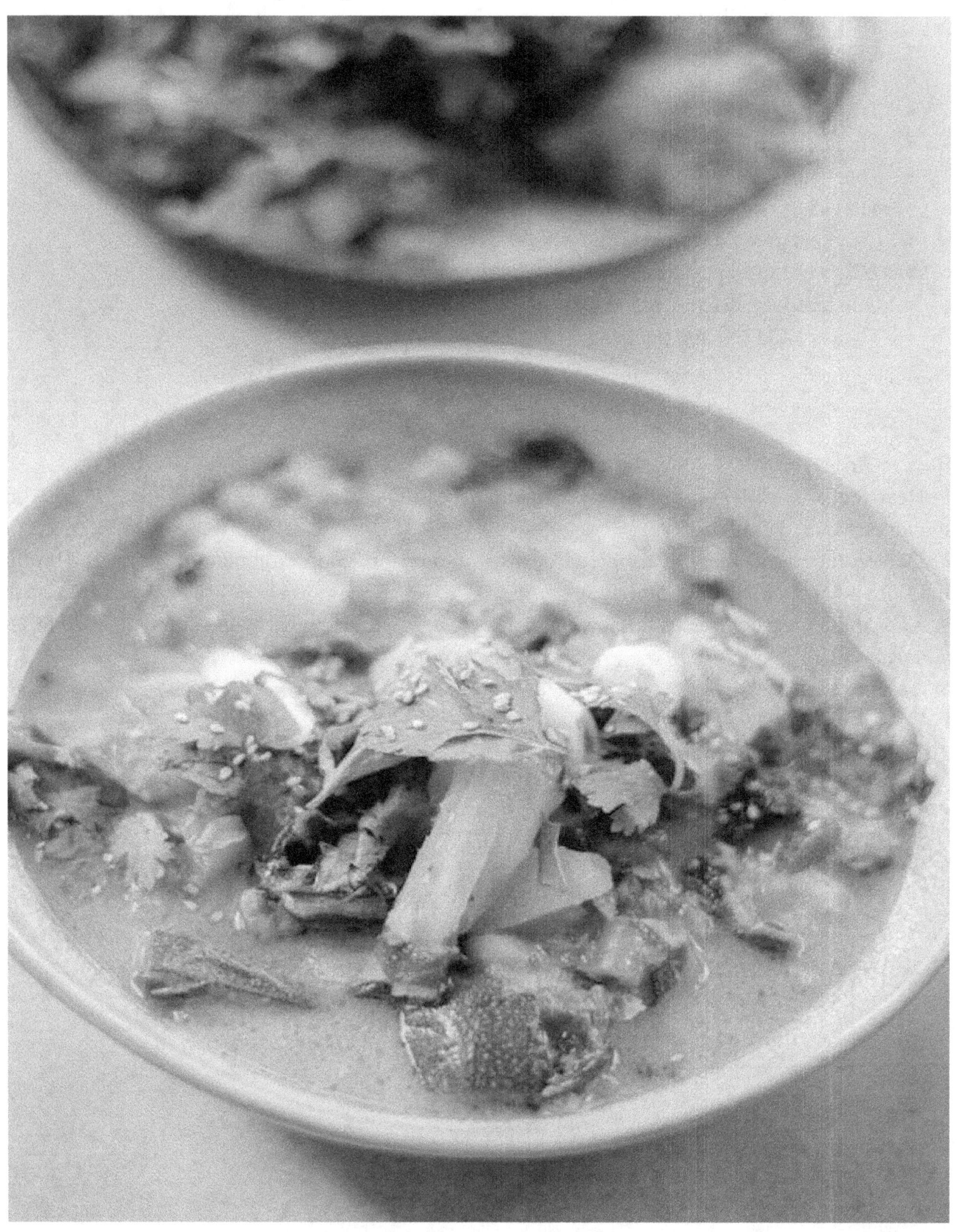

Ingredients:

- 1 tablespoon olive oil
- 1 chopped onion
- 2 minced garlic cloves
- One sliced red bell pepper
- One sliced carrot
- One can (13.5 oz) milk from coconuts
- Four cups of reduced-sodium vegetable broth and two tablespoons of Thai red curry paste
- 1 tablespoon soy sauce (for a gluten-free substitute, use tamari).
- 1 tablespoon of coconut sugar (or brown sugar)
- One lime's juice
- To taste salt
- Chopped fresh cilantro (as a garnish)

How to Prepare:

1. Heat the olive oil in a big pot over medium heat. Diced onions, carrots, red bell pepper, and garlic should all be sautéed until tender.
2. Include the soy sauce, brown sugar, lime juice, coconut milk, vegetable broth, Thai red curry paste, and salt. Heat through to a simmer.
3. To allow the flavors to mingle, simmer for 15 to 20 minutes.
4. Before serving, garnish with finely chopped fresh cilantro.

Time Required for Preparation: 30 minutes

Nutritional Worth: When eaten in moderation, this rich and creamy soup is low in carbohydrates and packed with nutrients, making it a great choice for diabetic diets.

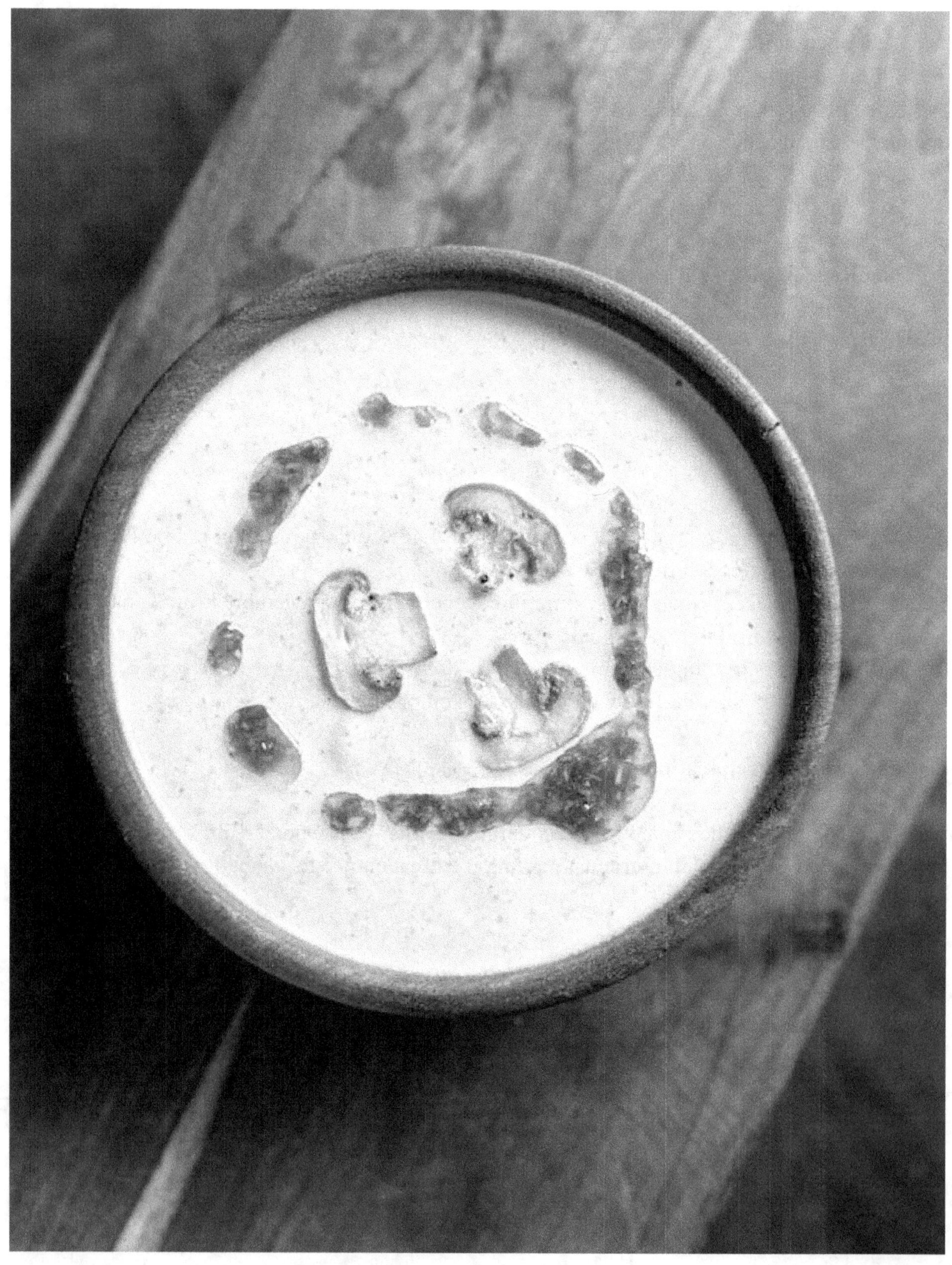

Ingredients:

- 1 tablespoon olive oil
- 1 chopped onion
- 2 chopped carrots
- Two chopped celery stalks
- Three minced garlic cloves
- 8 ounces of sliced mushrooms
- 1/2 cup of barley pearls
- One teaspoon dried thyme
- Six cups of low-sodium vegetable broth
- Adjust with salt and pepper to taste

Method of Preparation:

1. Heat the olive oil in a big pot over medium heat. Diced celery, carrots, onions, and garlic should be sautéed until tender.
2. Include the pearl barley and sliced mushrooms. Simmer for two to three minutes.
3. Add the dried thyme and pour in the vegetable broth. Heat till boiling.
4. Once the barley is soft, reduce heat and simmer for 45 to 50 minutes.
5. Before serving, add salt and pepper for seasoning.

Time Required for Preparation: 60 minutes

Value for Nutrition: This soup is a healthy choice for those with diabetes since it's high in fiber and a decent supply of complex carbs.

These soup recipes take into account the nutritional needs of those with diabetes while providing a range of flavors and nutrients. They help diabetics maintain stable blood sugar levels and general health since they are low in calories and carbohydrates and abundant in fiber, protein, and important vitamins and minerals.

CHAPTER 7

SNACKS RECIPES

Diabetic-friendly snack recipes, each with information on ingredients, preparation time, procedure, and nutritional value:

1. Berries with Greek Yogurt:

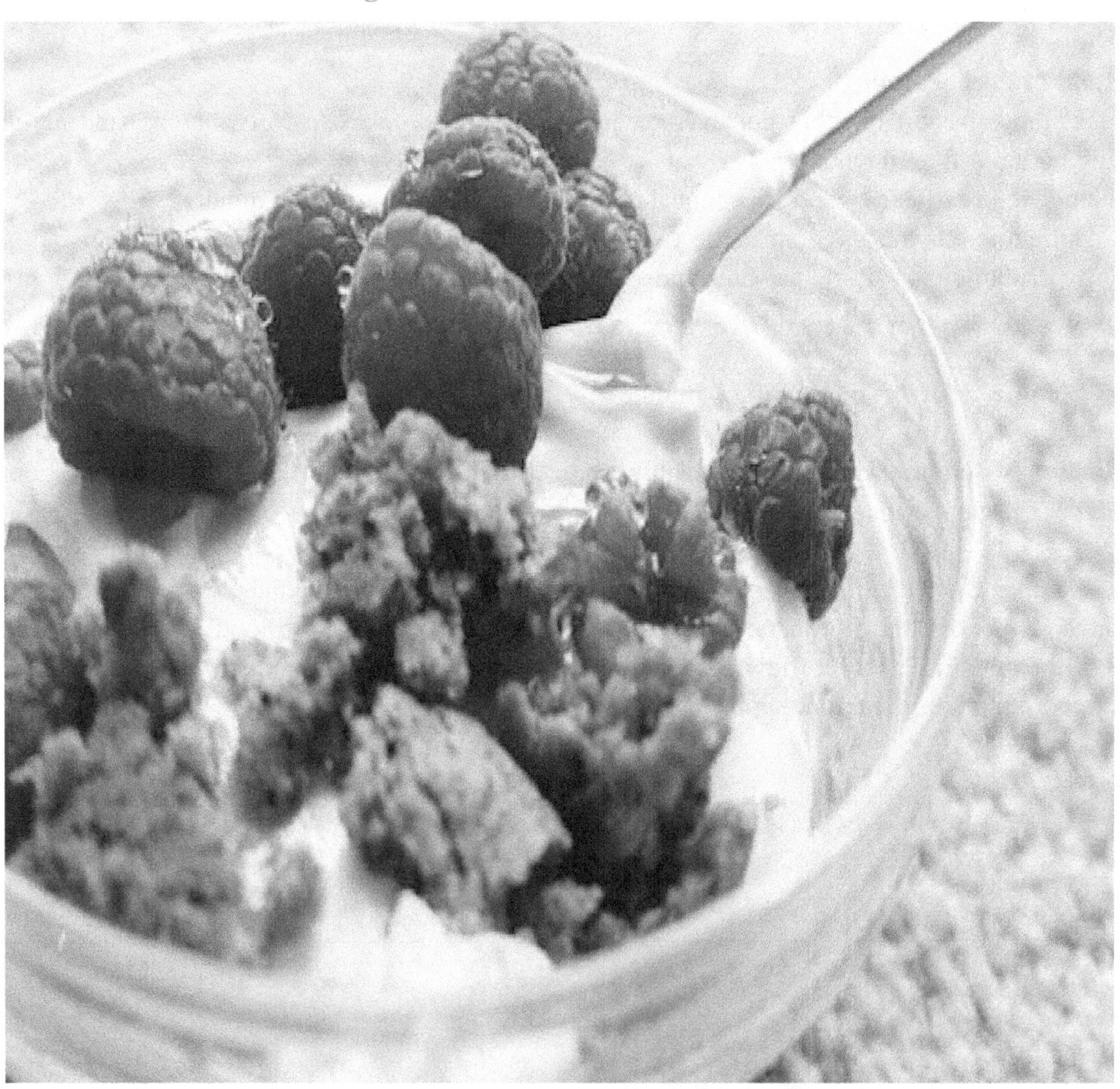

Ingredients:
- Half a cup of Greek yogurt
- One-fourth cup of assorted berries, including raspberries, blueberries, and strawberries
- One tablespoon of chopped nuts (walnuts, almonds, etc.)

How to Prepare:

Pour Greek yogurt into a bowl using a spoon.

2. Add chopped nuts and mixed berries on top.

3. Present right away.

Time Spent Preparing: Five minutes

Value for Nutrition: This food is excellent for regulating blood sugar levels because it is low in carbohydrates and high in protein, fiber, and antioxidants.

2. Hummus-topped vegetable sticks:

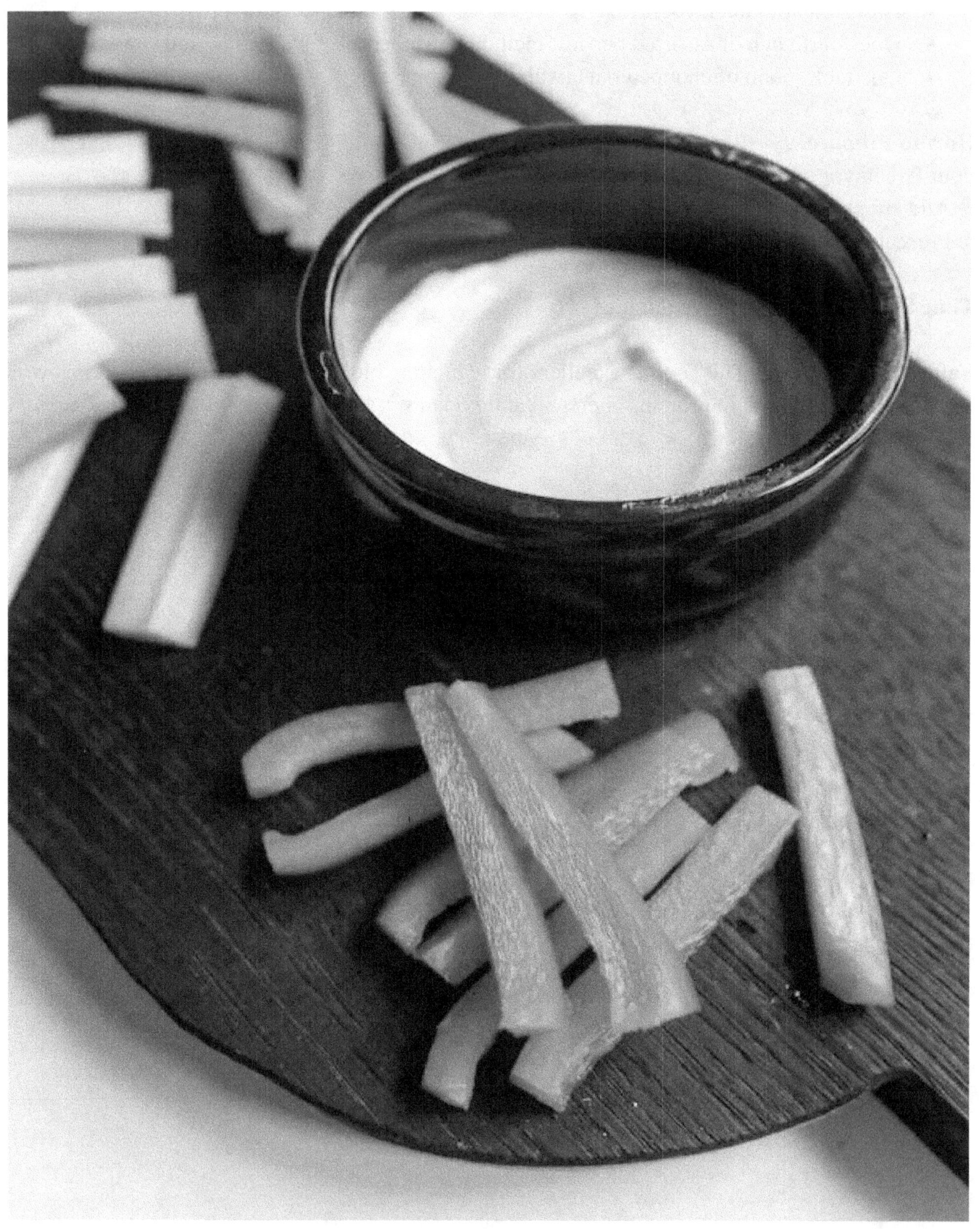

Ingredients:
- One carrot, thinly sliced
- One cucumber, thinly sliced
- One bell pepper, thinly sliced
- Two tablespoons of hummus

How to Prepare:
1. Put the veggie sticks on a platter.
2. Accompany with hummus for dunks.

Time Required for Preparation: 10 minutes

Value for Nutrition: This food, which is low in calories and carbohydrates and high in fiber, vitamins, and minerals, gives you long-lasting energy without raising your blood sugar.

3. Hard-Boiled Eggs with Avocado Slices:

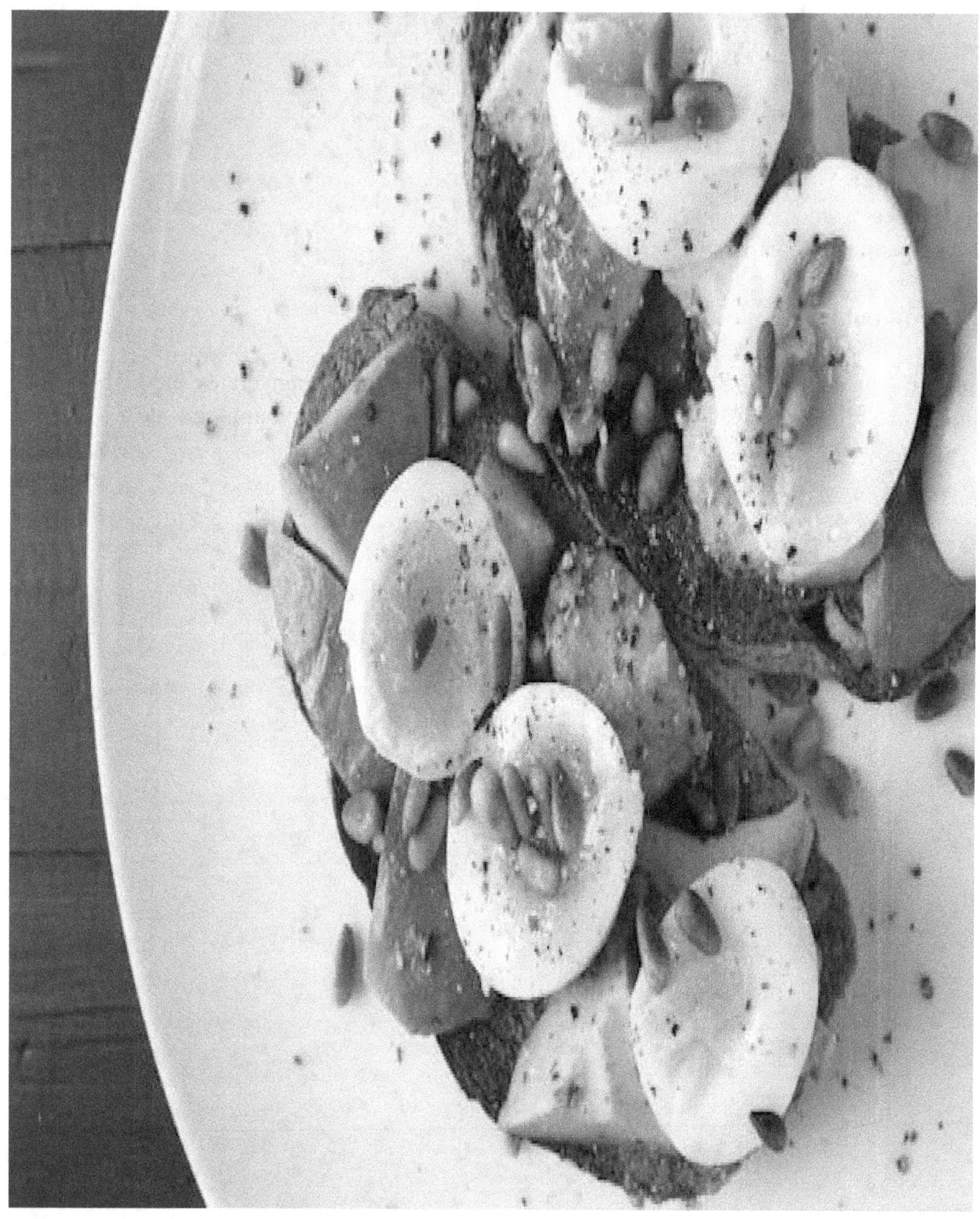

Ingredients:
- Two eggs, hard-boiled
- Half of an avocado, cut
- A dash of pepper and salt

Preparation Technique:
1. Hard-boiled eggs should be peeled and cut in half.
2. Put slices of avocado on a platter.
3. Top avocado slices with half of a hard-boiled egg.
4. Add a dash of pepper and salt for seasoning.

Time Required for Preparation: 15 minutes (boiling eggs included)

Value Nutritional: This snack is rich in fiber, healthy fats, and protein, which delivers vital nutrients and helps control blood sugar levels.

4. Pineapple Chunks with Cottage Cheese:

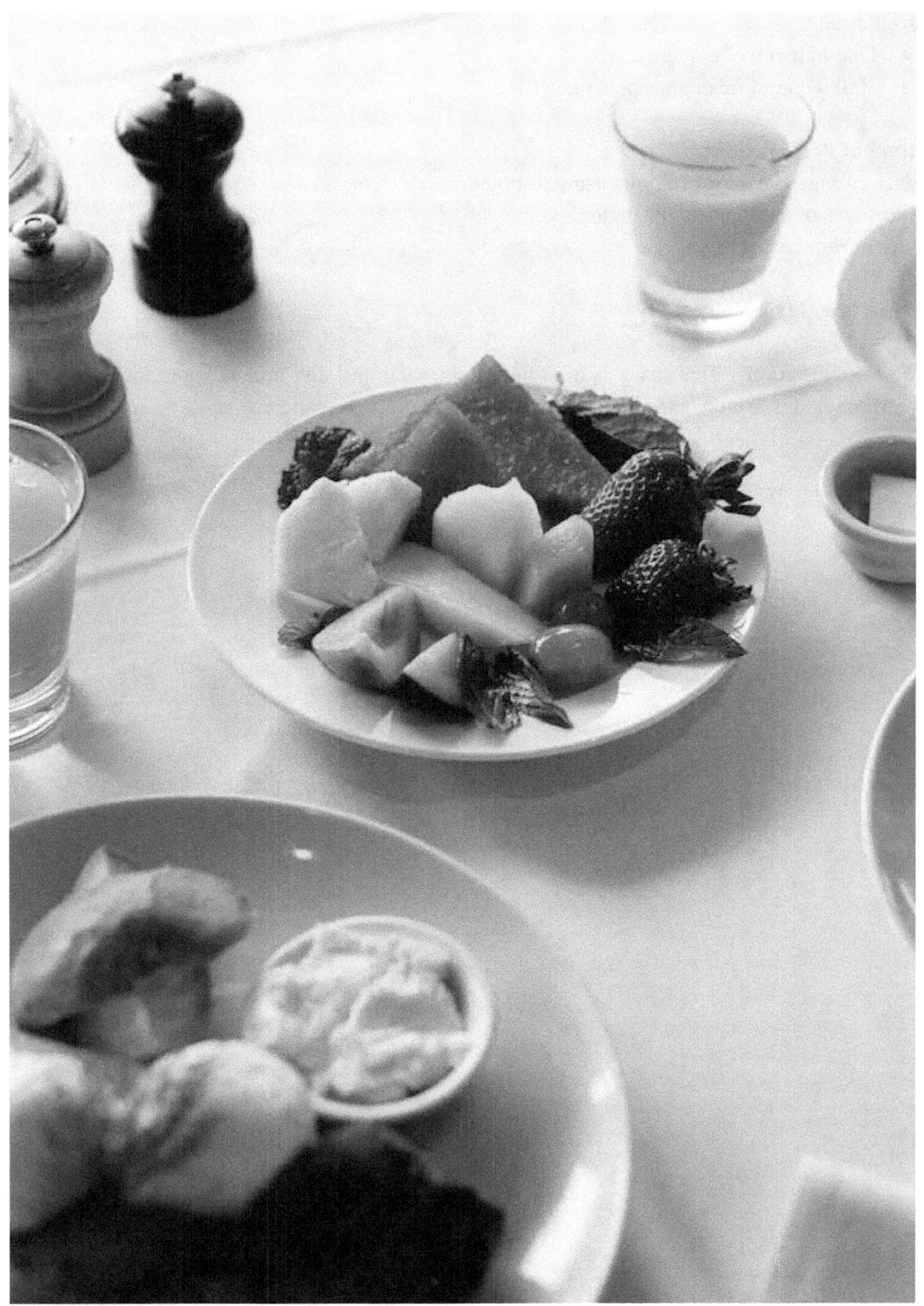

Ingredients:
- One-half cup of cottage cheese
- Half a cup of fresh pineapple pieces

Method of Preparation:
1. Place cottage cheese into a bowl using a spoon.
2. Add slices of fresh pineapple on top.
3. Present right away.

Set Up Time: Five minutes

Value for Nutrition: This snack is high in protein, vitamins, and minerals and low in calories and carbohydrates, which helps with blood sugar regulation and satiety.

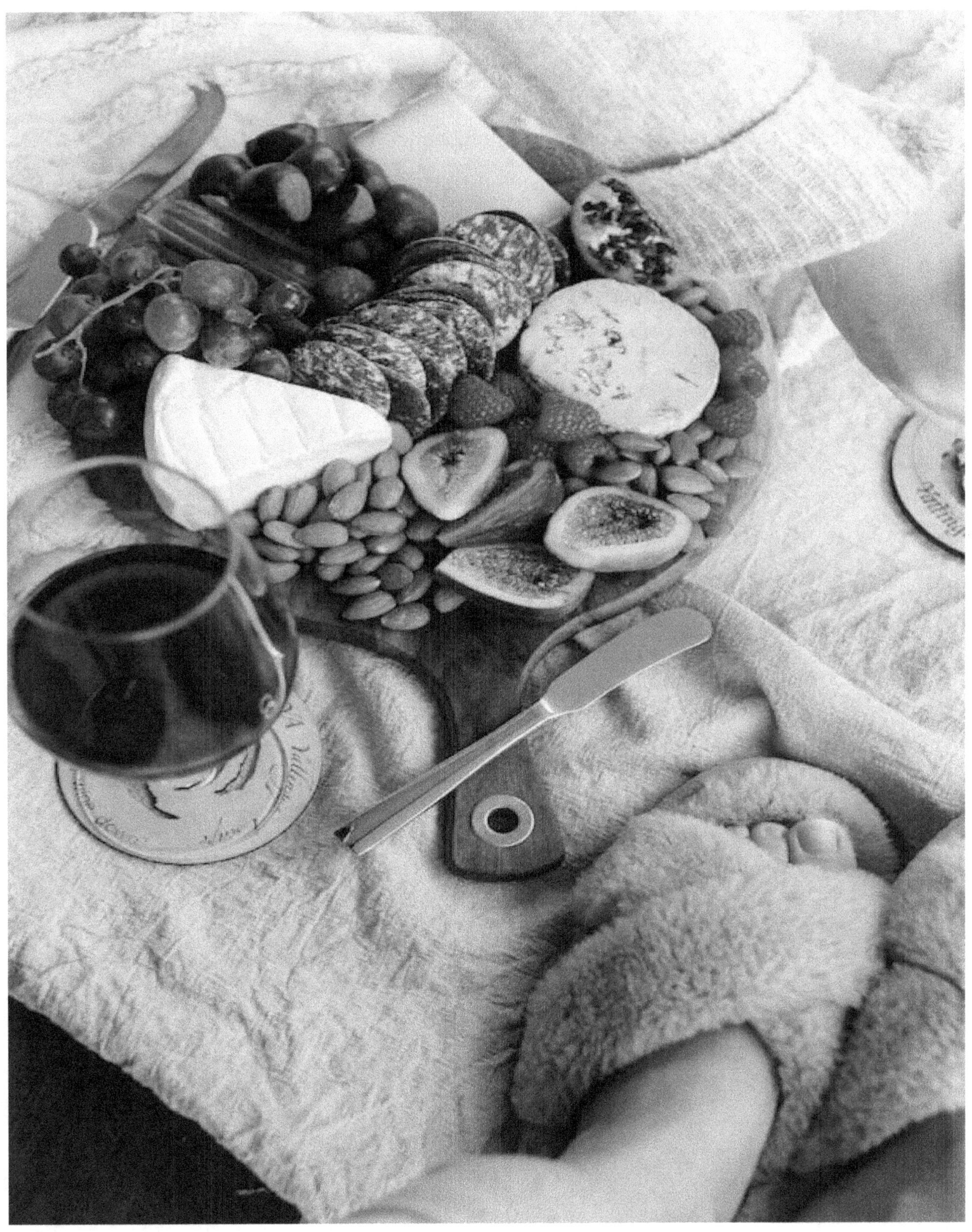

Ingredients:

- Two tablespoons of almond butter
- Four whole-grain crackers

Method of Preparation:

1. Evenly spread whole-grain crackers with almond butter.
2. Present right away.

Set Up Time: Five minutes

Value for Nutrition: This food helps control blood sugar levels and provides continuous energy. It is a wonderful dose of fiber, protein, and healthy fats.

6. Tuna Salad with Cucumber Rounds:

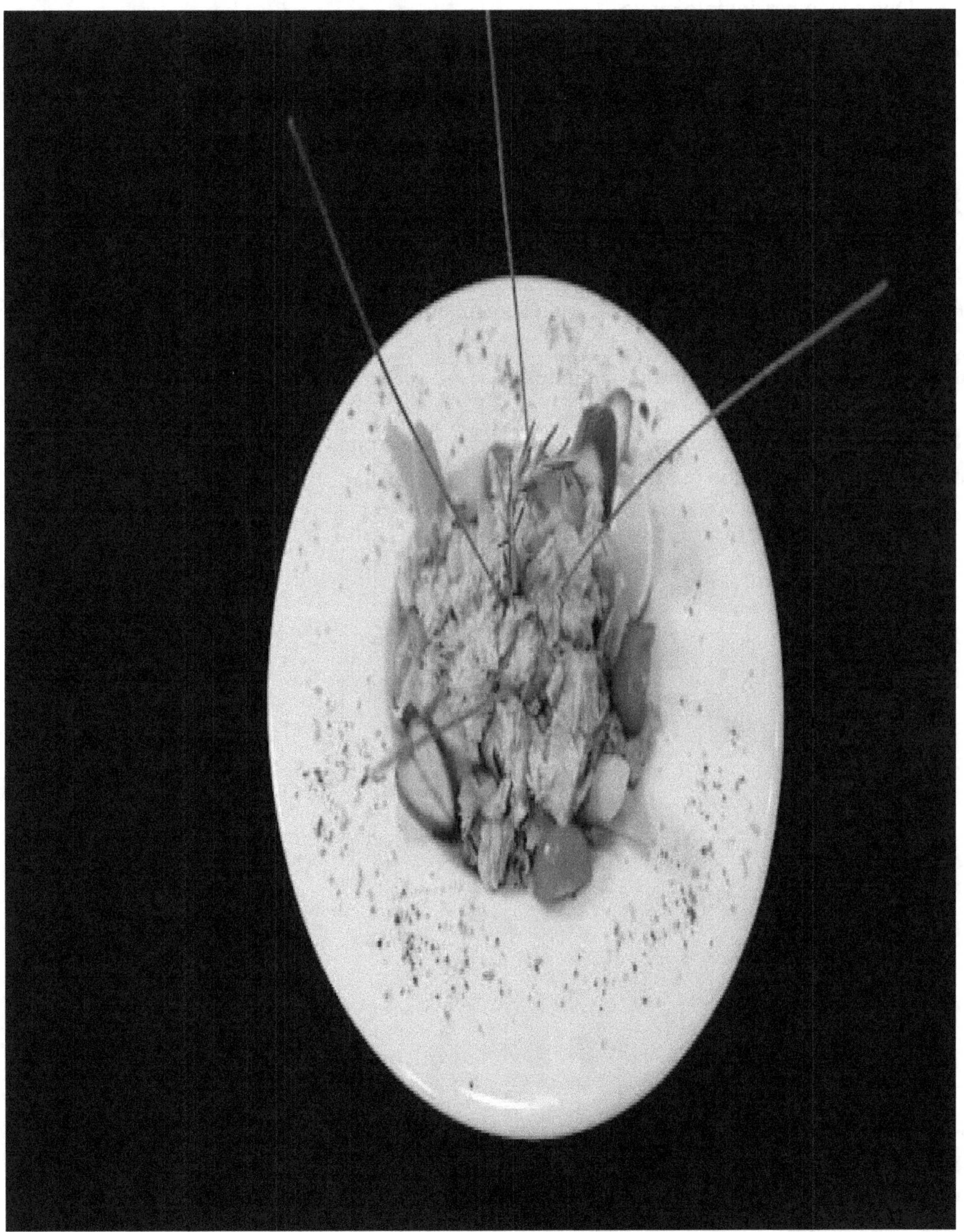

Ingredients:

- One cucumber cut into circles
- One can (5 oz) of drained tuna
- One tablespoon of mayonnaise (for a lighter option, use Greek yogurt)
- Half a tablespoon of mustard
- To taste, add salt and pepper.

How to Prepare:

1. Combine the drained tuna, mustard, mayonnaise, salt, and pepper in a bowl.
2. Arrange rounds of cucumber on a platter.
3. Place a dollop of tuna salad on top of each cucumber round.

Time Required for Preparation: 10 minutes

Value for Nutrition: This snack, which is low in carbohydrates and high in protein, gives vital nutrients and stabilizes blood sugar levels.

7. Salted Chickpeas:

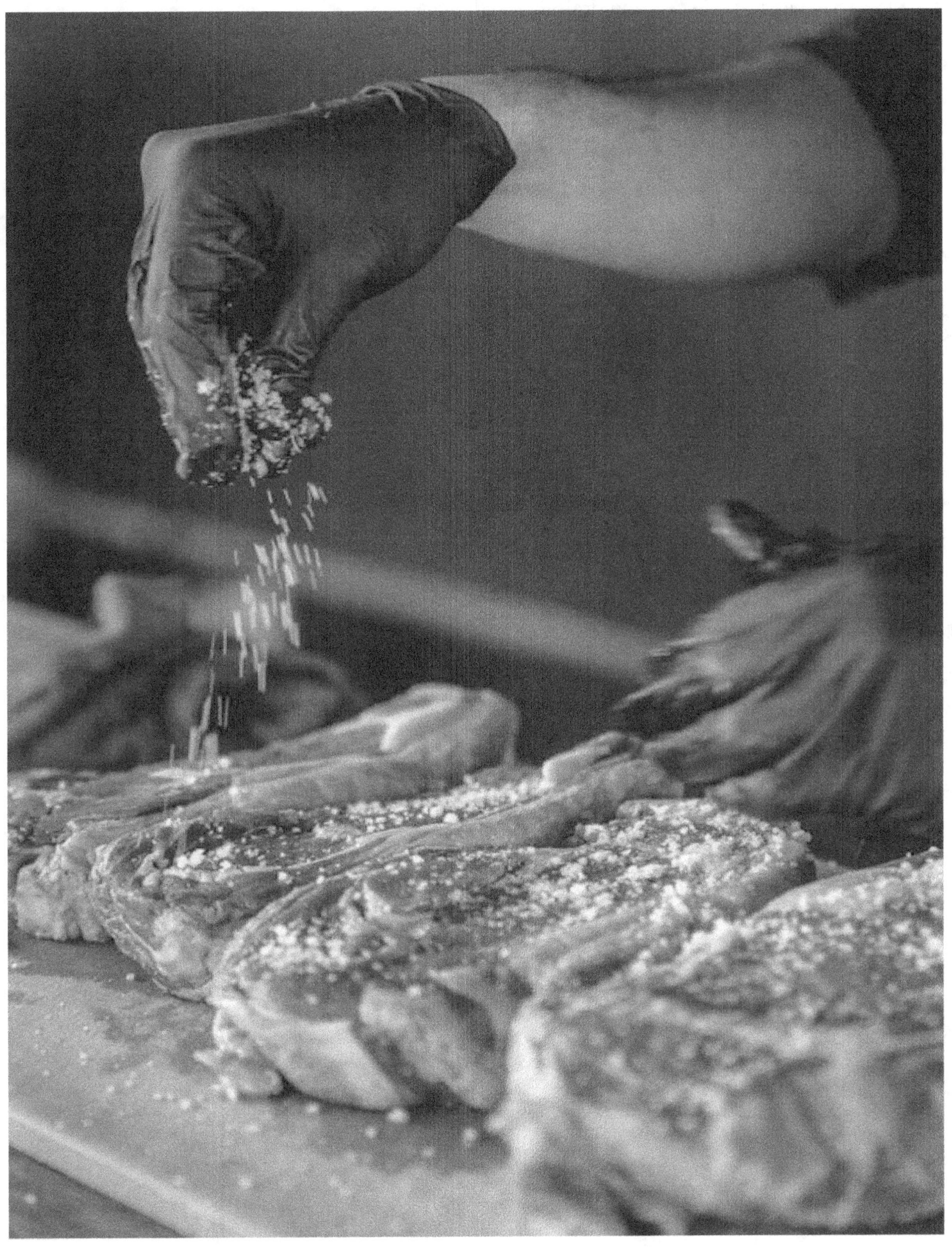

Substances:

- One 15-oz can of washed and drained chickpeas
- One tablespoon of olive oil
- One teaspoon ground cumin
- One teaspoon paprika
- 1/2 tsp. powdered garlic
- Salt according to taste

Method of Preparation:

1. Set oven temperature to 200°C/400°F.

2. Using a paper towel, pat dry the chickpeas to absorb any remaining moisture.

3. Toss the chickpeas in a bowl with the olive oil, salt, paprika, ground cumin, and garlic powder until well covered.

4. Arrange the chickpeas on a baking sheet in a single layer.

5. Roast, shaking the pan halfway through, for 25 to 30 minutes in a preheated oven, or until crispy.

6. Let cool completely before serving.

Set Up Time: thirty-five minutes

Value for Nutrition: Roasted chickpeas are a crispy snack high in protein and fiber that increases satiety and helps control blood sugar levels.

8. Peanut butter-topped apple slices:

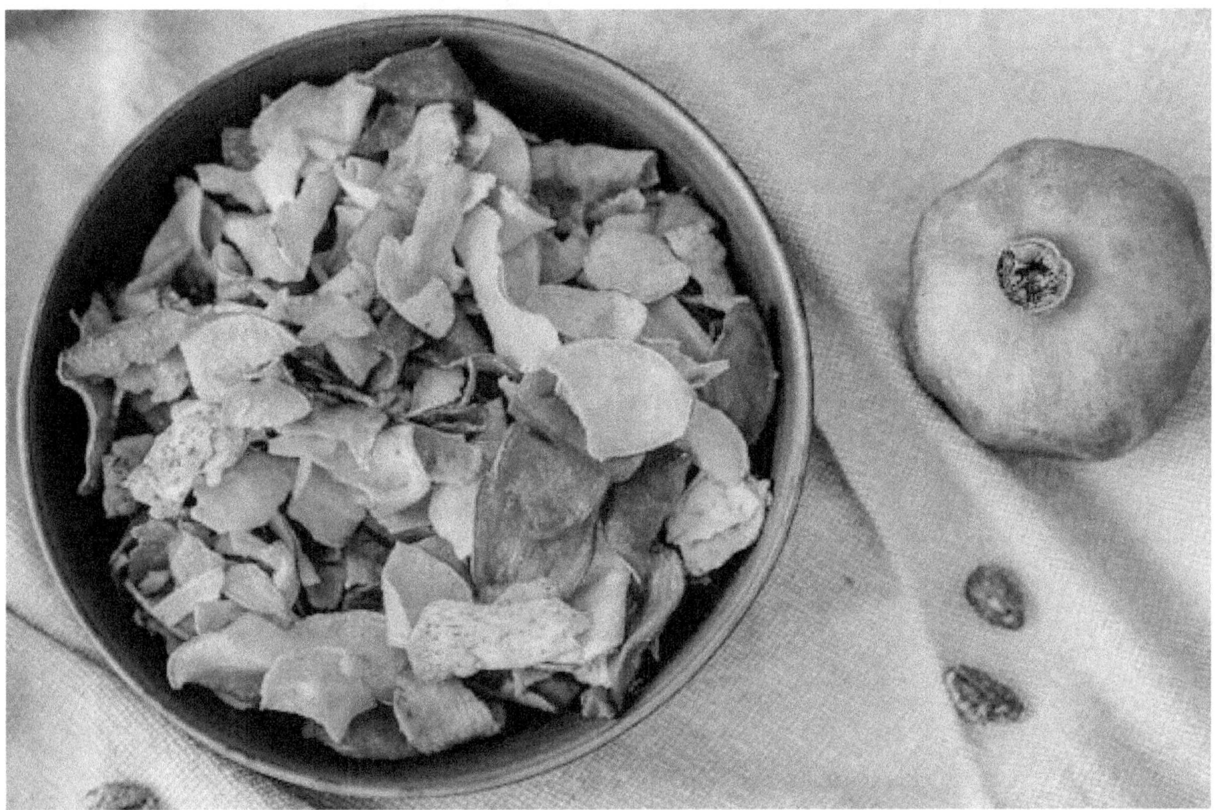

Ingredients:
- Two tablespoons of natural peanut butter without added sugar
- One medium apple, sliced

How to Prepare:
1. Arrange slices of apple on a platter.
2. Accompany with peanut butter for spreading or dipping.

Set Up Time: Five minutes

Value for Nutrition: This snack offers vital nutrients and a balance of healthy fats, carbohydrates, and protein, helping to maintain stable blood sugar levels.

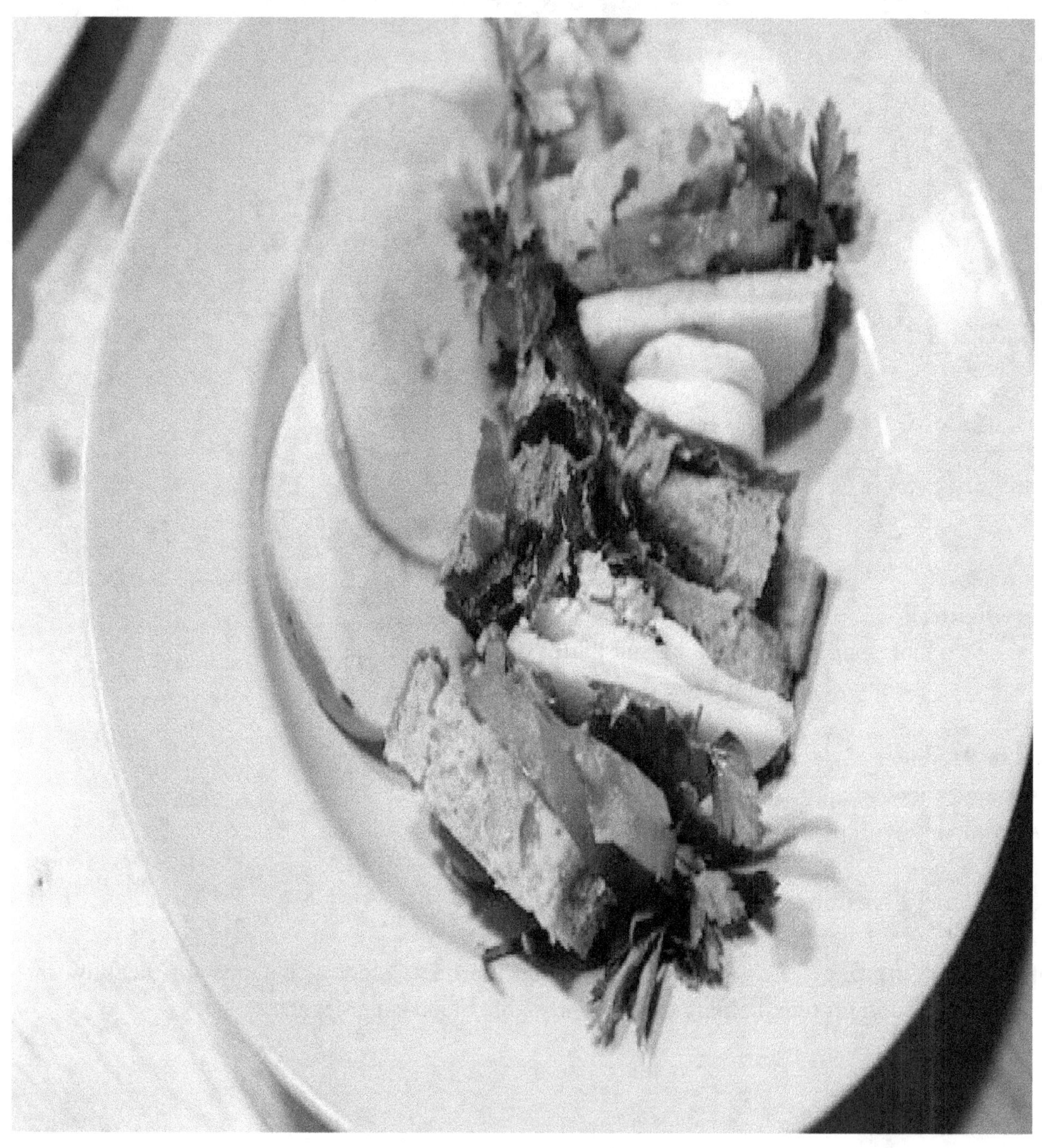

Ingredients:
- Four chopped celery stalks
- One ounce of smoked salmon
- Two tablespoons of cream cheese (for a lighter option, use Greek yogurt cream cheese).

How to Prepare:
1. Evenly coat celery sticks with cream cheese.
2. Place a piece of smoked salmon on top of every celery stick.

Time Spent Preparing: 10 minutes

Crucial Point: This food, which is high in protein, vitamins, and omega-3 fatty acids, promotes blood sugar regulation and heart health.

10. Sea Salt Edamame:

Ingredients:
- One cup of edamame, either fresh or frozen; sea salt to taste

Method of Preparation:
1. If using frozen edamame, cook or steam it until it becomes soft, following the directions on the package.
2. To make fresh edamame tender, steam or boil them for five to seven minutes.
3. After draining, toss the cooked edamame with sea salt.
4. You can serve it cold or heated.

Time Required for Preparation: 10 minutes

Value for Nutrition: Edamame is a healthy snack choice for those with diabetes because it's high in protein, fiber, and other important nutrients.

These snack dishes provide vital nutrients and help diabetics control their blood sugar levels, all while showcasing a diversity of flavors and textures.

CHAPTER 8

DESSERT RECIPES

Dessert recipes that are appropriate for people with diabetes, along with information on ingredients, preparation time, method, and nutritional value:

1. Compounded Berries Parfait:

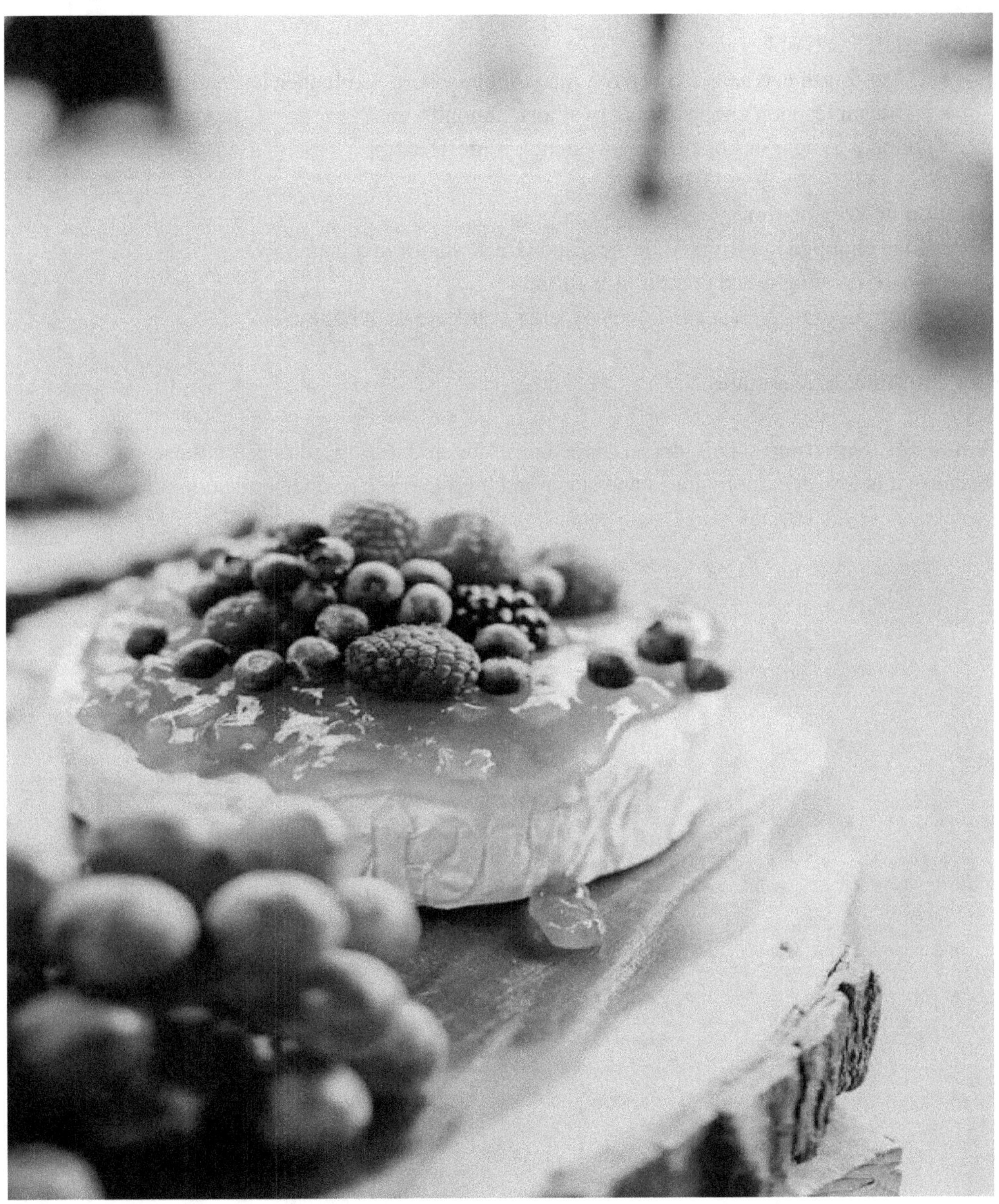

Constituents:

- Half a cup of Greek yogurt
- One-fourth cup assorted berries, including raspberries, blueberries, and strawberries
- One tablespoon chopped nuts (walnuts, almonds, etc.)
- One tsp sugar or honey-free sweetener, if preferred

Method of Preparation:

1. Arrange chopped nuts, mixed berries, and Greek yogurt in a glass.
2. Continue layering the glass until it is full.
3. If preferred, top with a sugar-free sweetener or drizzle with honey.

Set Up Time: Five minutes

Value for Nutrition: This dessert is a nutritious and filling choice for those with diabetes because it is low in carbohydrates and sugar and high in protein, fiber, and antioxidants.

2. Strawberries Covered in Dark Chocolate:

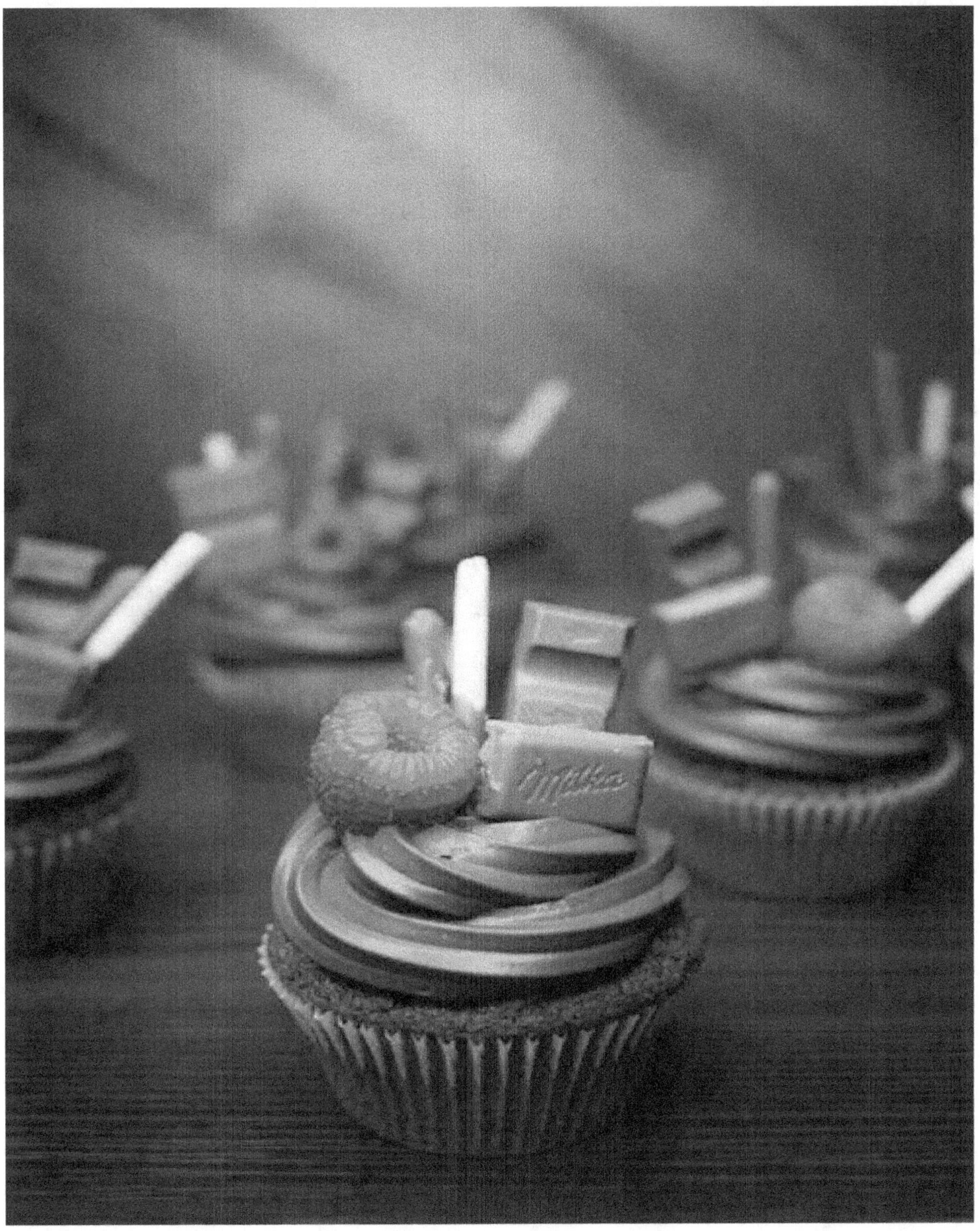

Ingredients:
- huge strawberries
- One ounce of melted dark chocolate (70% cocoa or higher)

Method of Preparation:
1. Thoroughly wash and pat dry strawberries.
2. Coat around two-thirds of each strawberry with melted dark chocolate by dipping it in.
3. Transfer to a baking sheet covered with parchment paper and chill until the chocolate solidifies.

Time Required for Preparation: 15 minutes

Value for Nutrition: Because dark chocolate has more antioxidants and less sugar than milk chocolate, combined with strawberries' low calorie and carb content, this dessert can be enjoyed in moderation by those with diabetes.

3. Cinnamon-Baked Apples:

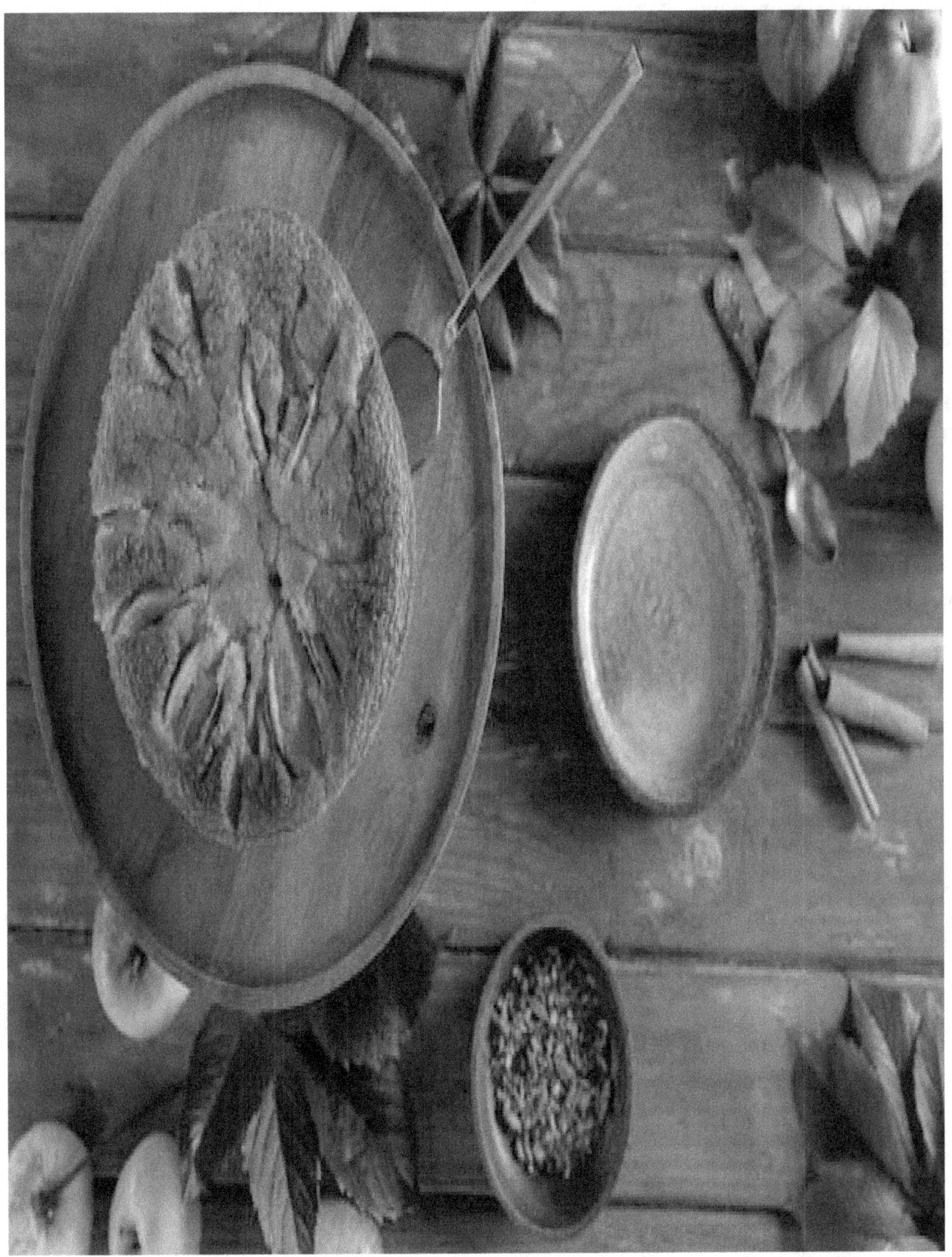

Ingredients:

- Two apples, medium
- One teaspoon of cinnamon
- Half a teaspoon of nutmeg
- One tablespoon of chopped nuts (walnuts, pecans, etc.)
- One tsp sugar or honey-free sweetener, if preferred

How to Prepare:

1. Set oven temperature to 175°C/350°F.
2. Core the apples and cut them lengthwise in half.
3. Put the cut sides of the apple halves in a baking dish.
4. Dust the apples with nutmeg and cinnamon.
5. Bake apples for 20 to 25 minutes, or until they are soft.
6. Top baked apples with chopped nuts and honey, or top with sugar-free sweetener if preferred.

Time Required for Preparation: half an hour

Value for Nutrition: Because apples are high in vitamins and fiber and because cinnamon may help lower blood sugar, this dessert is a good choice for those with diabetes.

4. Chia Seed Pudding:

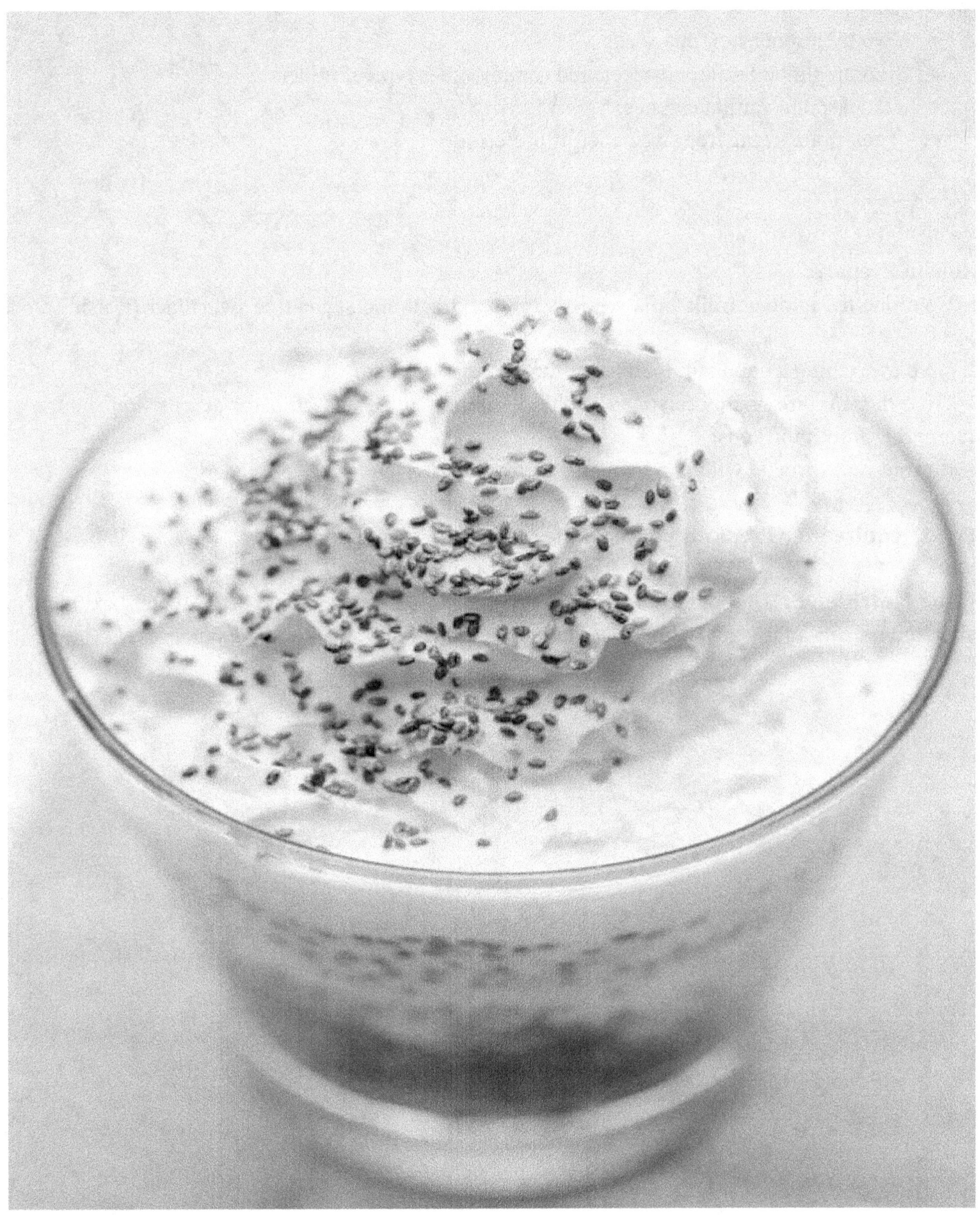

Ingredients

- Two tablespoons of chia seeds
- 1/2 cup almond milk, unsweetened (or any other type of milk)
- 1/4 teaspoon vanilla essence;
- 1 teaspoon sugar-free sweetener, if preferred

How to Prepare:

1. Combine the almond milk, chia seeds, vanilla extract, and sugar-free sweetener (if using) in a bowl.
2. Give everything a good stir, then leave for five minutes.
3. Give the mixture one more stir to avoid clumping, cover, and chill for at least four hours, or overnight, until it thickens.
4. If preferred, sprinkle with chopped nuts or fresh berries and serve chilled.

Time Required for Preparation: 5 minutes (including cooling period)

Value Nutritional: This dessert is perfect for diabetics because chia seeds, which are high in fiber and omega-3 fatty acids, provide vital nutrients without raising blood sugar levels.

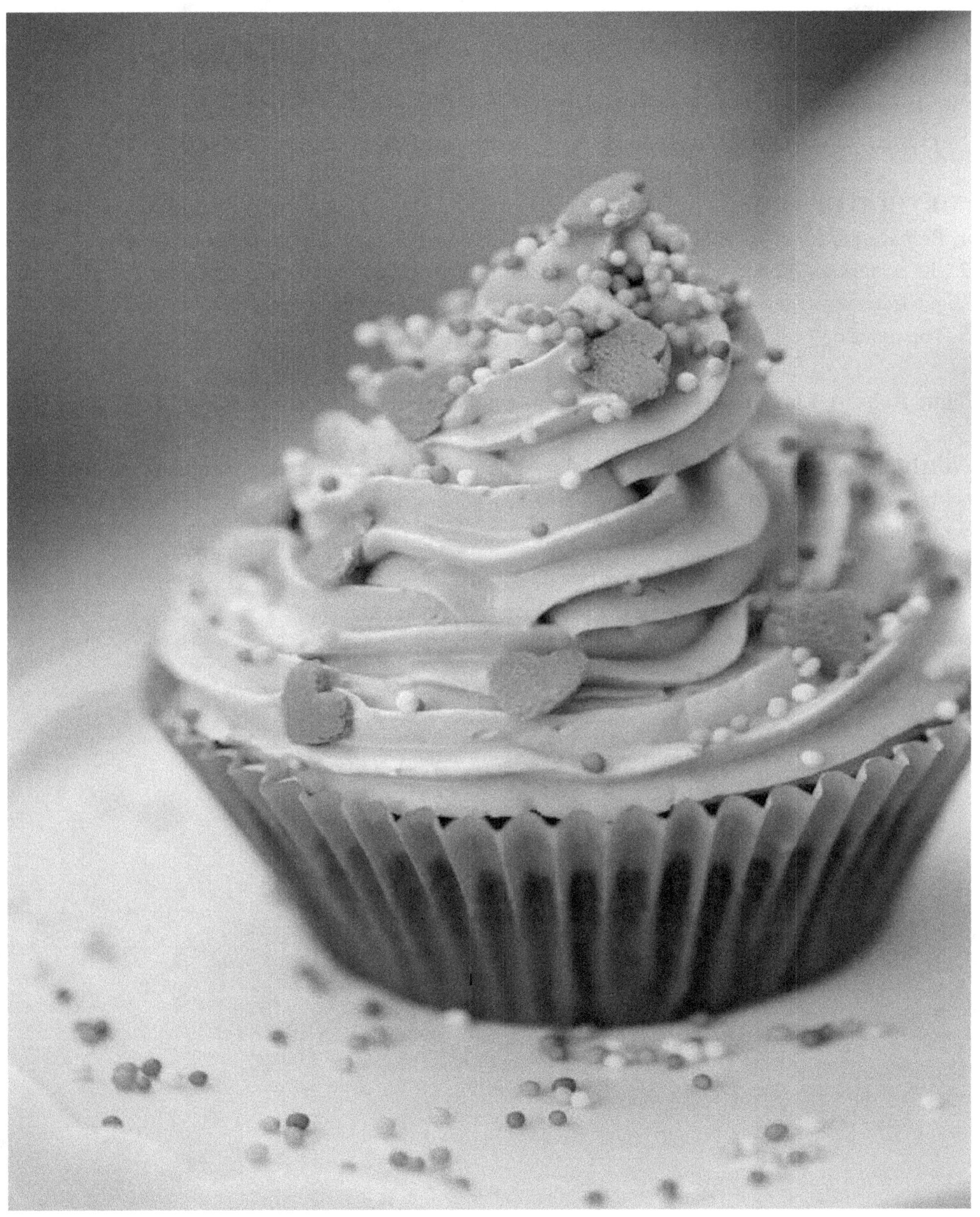

Ingredients:
One package (any flavor) of sugar-free Jello
Half a cup of thickened cream
One teaspoon of vanilla extract
Sweetener without added sugar, to taste

METHOD OF PREP:
1. Prepare the sugar-free Jello per the directions on the package, then refrigerate to set.
2. In a another bowl, beat heavy cream until firm peaks form, adding vanilla extract and sugar-free sweetener.
3. Top a dollop of whipped cream with sugar-free Jello.

Time Required for Preparation: Two hours (including Jello setting time)

Nutritional Value: Sugar-free Jello is low in calories and carbohydrates, and when combined with homemade heavy cream whipped cream, it makes a delectable and filling dessert for those with diabetes.

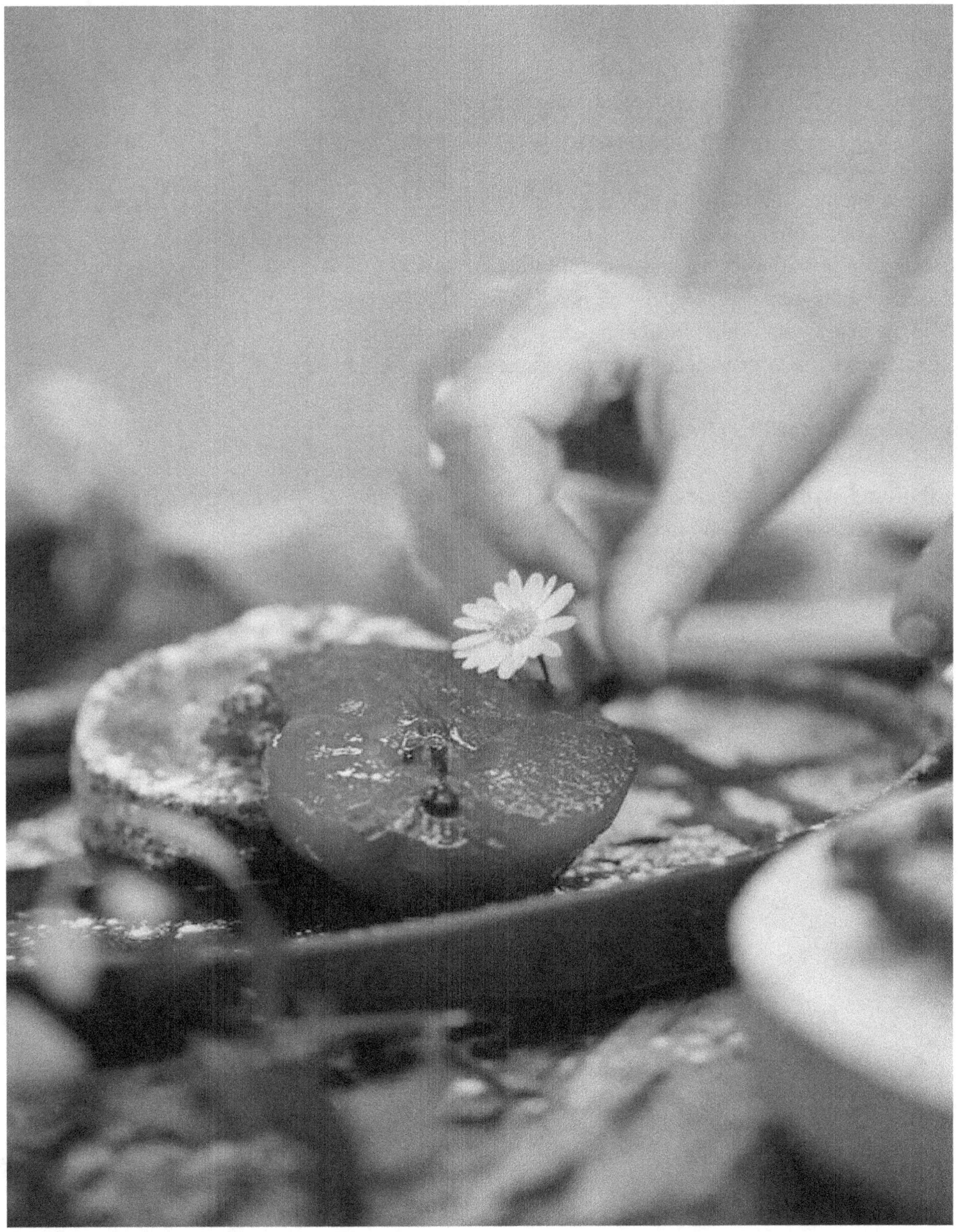

Ingredients:
- 1 tablespoon chopped nuts (almonds, pistachios)
- 1/4 cup ricotta cheese
- 2 ripe pears, cut in half and cored
- One tsp sugar or honey-free sweetener, if preferred

How to Prepare:
1. Set oven temperature to 190°C/375°F.
2. Put the cut-side-up pears in a casserole for baking.
3. Bake pears for 20 to 25 minutes, or until they are soft.
4. Place a tablespoon of ricotta cheese inside each half of a pear.
5. Top the pears with ricotta filling and chopped almonds.
6. If preferred, top with a sugar-free sweetener or drizzle with honey.

Time Required for Preparation: 30 minutes

Nutritional Worth: This dessert is a healthy and diabetic-friendly choice because pears are high in fiber and antioxidants and ricotta cheese adds protein and calcium.

7. Chocolate Mousse with Avocado:

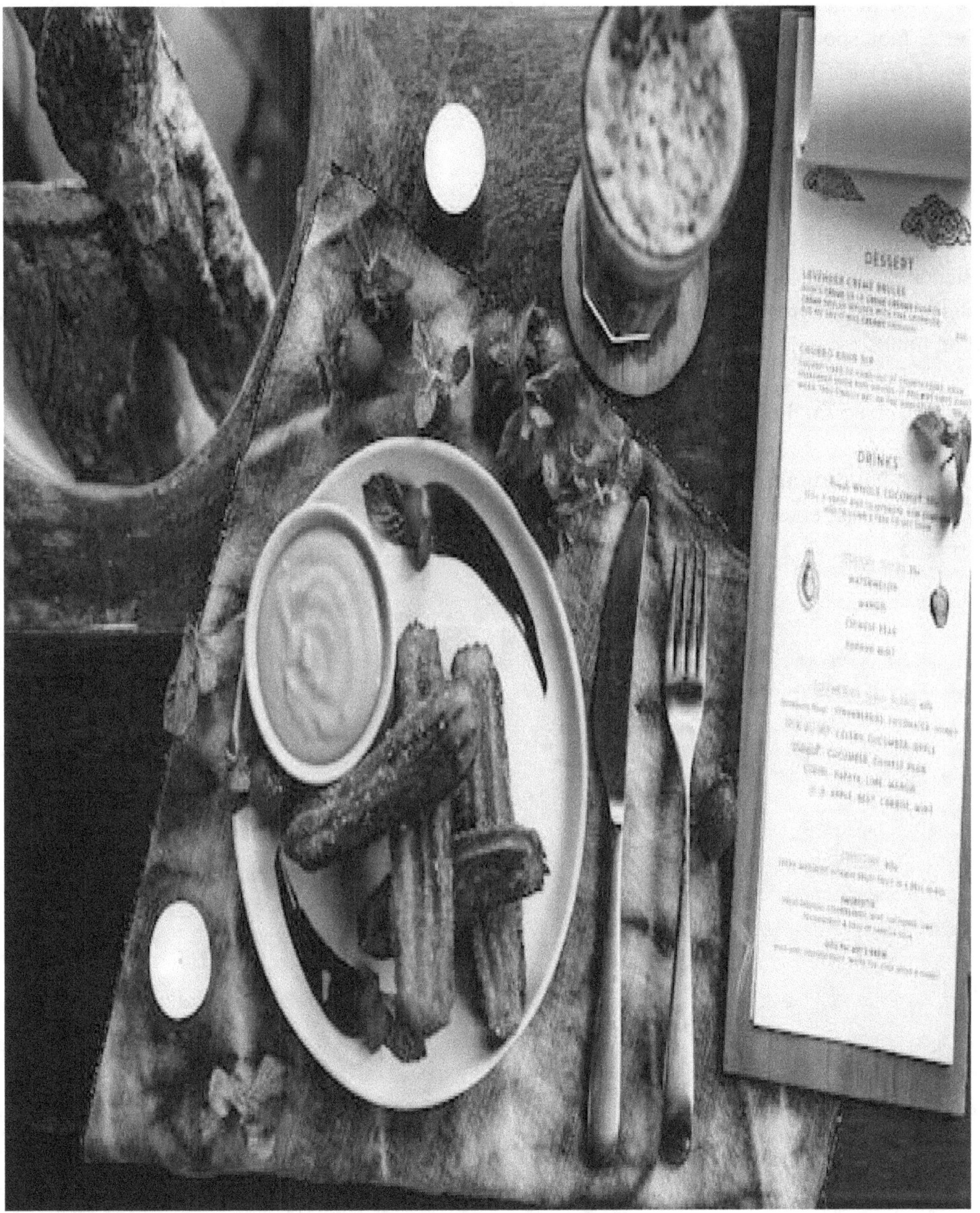

Ingredients:
- One mature avocado
- 2 tablespoons unsweetened cocoa powder
- Two tablespoons of sugarless sweetener (erythritol or stevia)
- One-half teaspoon vanilla extract

How to Prepare:
1. Remove the avocado's flesh with a spoon and transfer it to a food processor or blender.
2. Fill the blender with vanilla extract, sugar-free sweetener, and chocolate powder.
3. Blend, scraping down the sides as necessary, until creamy and smooth.
4. Before serving, transfer the mousse to serving dishes and let it cool in the fridge for at least half an hour.

Time Required for Preparation: 10 minutes (including cooling period)

Value for Nutrition: Avocado is a good source of fiber and healthy fats, and this dessert is excellent for diabetics because cocoa powder adds flavor and antioxidants without adding extra sugar.

8. Pineapple Macaroons:

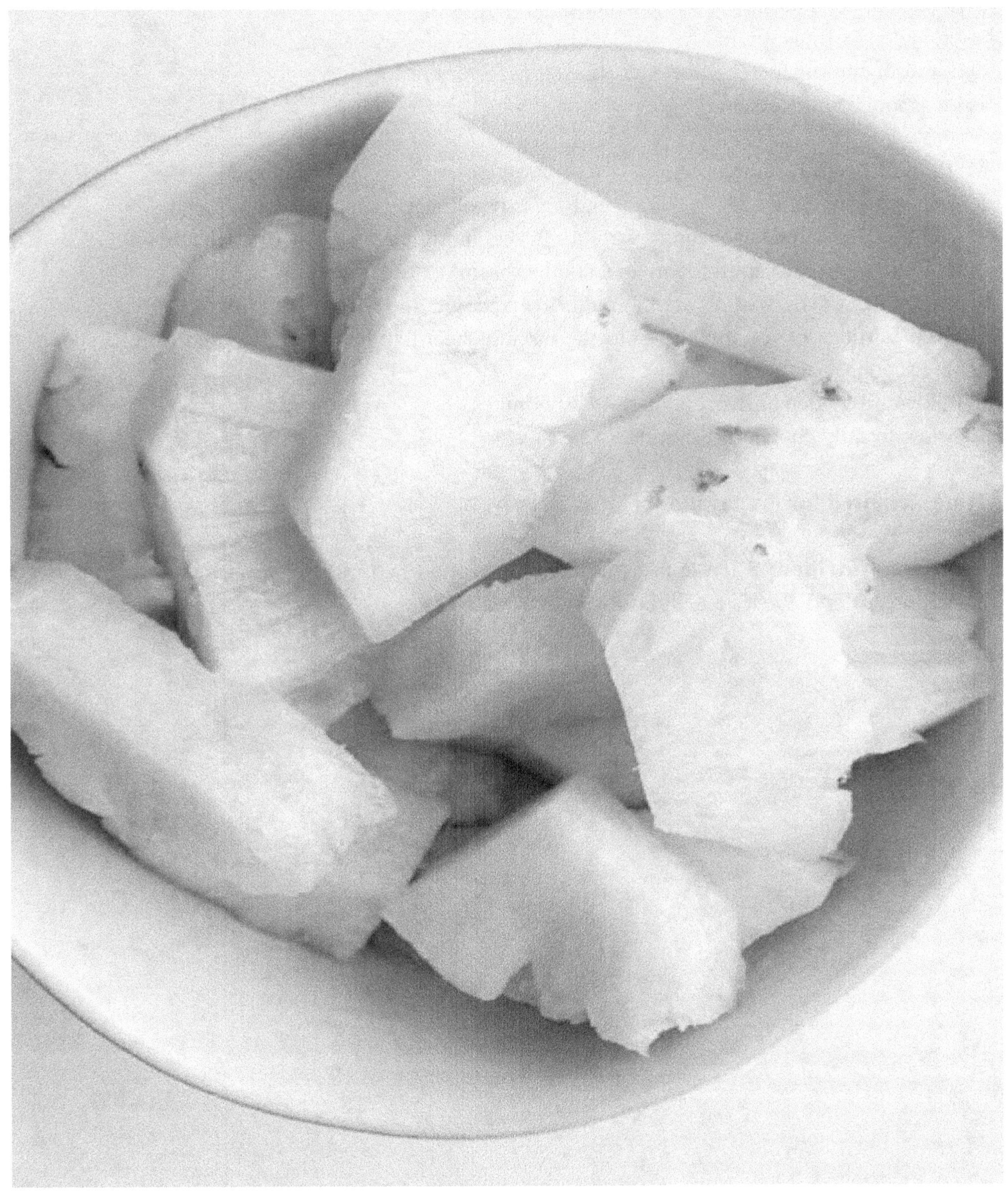

Constitution:
Two cups of coconut shreds without sugar
 Two big egg whites
One-fourth cup sugar-free sweetener (like stevia or erythritol)
1/4 teaspoon vanilla essence

Method of Preparation:
1. Preheat the oven to 325°F (160°C) and place parchment paper on a baking pan.
2. Combine the shredded coconut, vanilla extract, and sugar-free sweetener in a bowl.
3. Beat the egg whites until foamy in a another basin.
4. Ensure that the egg whites are thoroughly mixed with the coconut mixture.
5. Drop portions of the mixture onto the baking sheet that has been prepared using a spoon or cookie scoop.
6. Bake until golden brown, about 18 to 20 minutes.
7. Allow to fully cool before cutting.

Time Required for Preparation: half an hour

Value for Nutrition: Rich in heart-healthy lipids and low in carbohydrates and sugar, coconut macaroons offer diabetics a delightfully sweet treat.

9. Pumpkin Chia Seed Pudding:

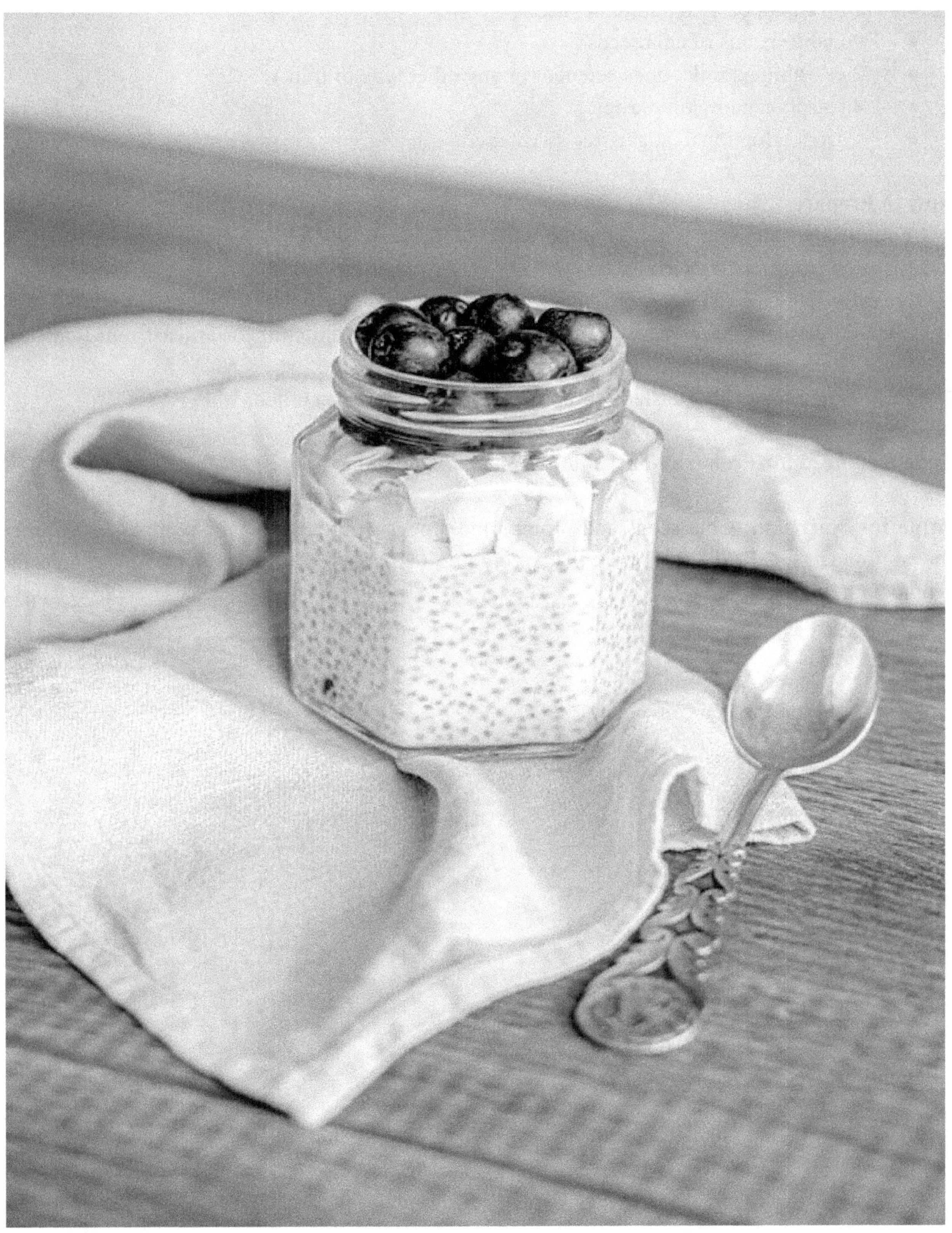

Ingredients:

- Half a cup of canned pumpkin puree
- Two tablespoons of chia seeds
- 1/2 cup almond milk, unsweetened (or any other type of milk)
- 1/4 teaspoon pumpkin pie spice
- 1 teaspoon (optional) sugar-free sweetener

How to Prepare:

1. Combine the pumpkin puree, almond milk, chia seeds, pumpkin pie spice, and sugar-free sweetener (if using) in a bowl.
2. Give everything a good stir, then leave for five minutes.
3. Give the mixture one more stir to avoid clumping, cover, and chill for at least four hours, or overnight, until it thickens.
4. If desired, garnish with a dash of pumpkin pie spice and serve chilled.

Time Required for Preparation: 5 minutes (including cooling period)

Value for Nutrition: Chia seeds add protein and omega-3 fatty acids, and pumpkin adds fiber and antioxidants. All of these ingredients combine to make this dessert a healthy choice for people with diabetes.

10. Yogurt Bark, Frozen:

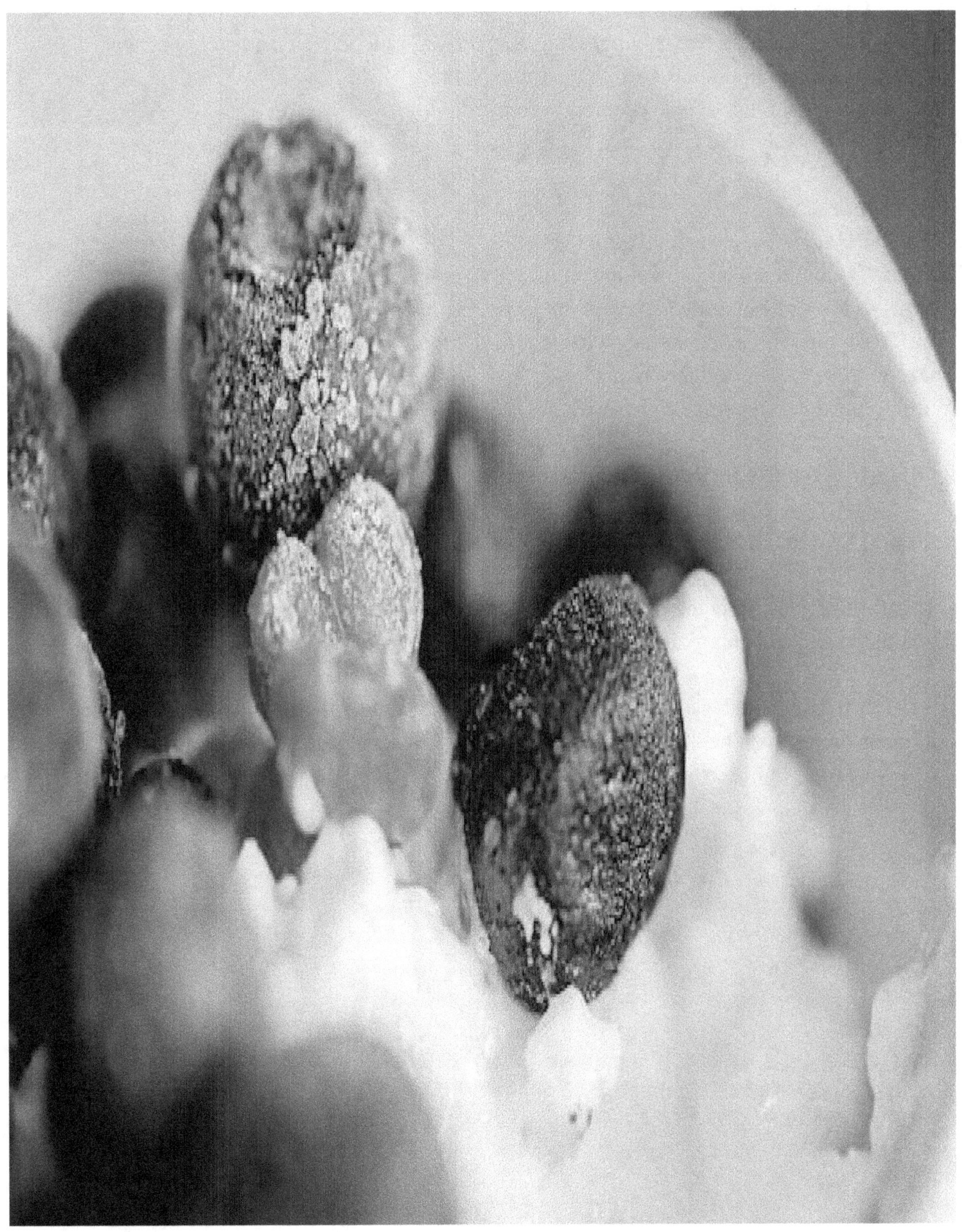

Contents:
One cup of Greek yogurt
One-fourth cup of assorted berries, including raspberries, blueberries, and strawberries
One tablespoon of chopped nuts (walnuts, almonds, etc.)
One tablespoon of shredded unsweetened coconut
One tsp sugar or honey-free sweetener, if preferred

How to Prepare:
1. Spread parchment paper over a baking sheet.
2. Using a 1/4-inch thick layer, evenly spread the Greek yogurt onto the parchment paper.
3. Top the yogurt with shredded coconut, chopped almonds, and mixed berries.
4. If preferred, top with a sugar-free sweetener or drizzle with honey.
5. Freeze until solid, two to three hours.
6. Split into portions and serve right away.

Time Required for Preparation: 10 minutes (including freezing time)

Nutritional Worth: Greek yogurt has a lot of protein.

low in carbohydrates, and the addition of fiber and antioxidants from the berries makes this dessert a nutritious and energizing choice for people with diabetes.

For those with diabetes, these dessert dishes provide delectable ways to indulge their sweet tooth without sacrificing their health. For individualized nutritional guidance, always seek the advice of a medical expert or dietician.

CHAPTER 9

<u>**30 DAYS MEAL PLAN**</u>

A 30-day diet plan for a novice with recently diagnosed diabetes:

Day 1:

Greek yogurt with berries and almonds for breakfast.
Lunch consists of grilled chicken salad topped with cucumber, tomato, and vinaigrette dressing on mixed greens.
Supper is baked salmon over quinoa and roasted asparagus.

Day 2:

Whole-grain toast served with a spinach and feta omelet for breakfast.
Lunch consists of lettuce, tomato, and an avocado and turkey wrap.
Brown rice, broccoli, and bell peppers with stir-fried tofu for dinner.

Day 3:

Breakfast: Oats, almond milk, chia seeds, and sliced strawberries on top of overnight oats.
Lentil soup and mixed green salad for lunch.
Steamed green beans and sweet potato with baked chicken breast for dinner.

Day 4:

Smoothie made with protein powder, banana, almond milk, and spinach for breakfast.
Quinoa salad and grilled shrimp skewers for lunch.
Brown rice noodles and vegetables stir-fried with tofu for dinner.

Day 5:

 Whole-grain bread and scrambled eggs with sautéed mushrooms for breakfast.
Greek salad with grilled chicken and whole-wheat pita for lunch.
Dinner is cauliflower rice, roasted Brussels sprouts, and baked cod.

Day 6:

Peach slices and a dash of cinnamon over cottage cheese for breakfast.
Brown rice stir-fried with turkey and vegetables for lunch.
Quinoa pilaf with grilled fish paired with steamed broccoli for dinner.

Day 7:

Waffles made with whole grains, topped with mixed berries and Greek yogurt for breakfast.
Chickpea salad with cucumbers, tomatoes, and feta cheese for lunch.
Supper is baked chicken thighs served over couscous and roasted carrots.

Day 8:

Vegetable scramble made with eggs, onions, bell peppers, and spinach for breakfast.
Tuna salad lettuce wraps with cherry tomatoes and avocado for lunch.
Dinner consists of marinara sauced turkey meatballs over zucchini noodles.

Day 9:

Protein shake for breakfast, consisting of protein powder, banana, spinach, and almond milk.
Lunch consists of a salad of quinoa, black beans, chopped avocado, and lime vinaigrette.
Wild rice with grilled shrimp paired with roasted vegetables for dinner.

Day 10:

Greek yogurt parfait with granola and strawberries cut into pieces for breakfast.
Lunch consists of mixed greens and a grilled vegetable wrap with hummus.
Brown rice stir-fried with beef and broccoli for dinner

Day 11:

Whole-grain toast with scrambled eggs, spinach, and mushrooms for breakfast.
Lunch consists of a salad of spinach and quinoa dressed with balsamic vinaigrette, grilled chicken, and cherry tomatoes.
Supper consists of baked cod fillet served with barley pilaf and roasted Brussels sprouts.

Day 12:

Pineapple parfait with cottage cheese and chopped walnuts for breakfast.
Lunch consists of mixed green salad on the side and lentil and vegetable soup.
Dinner is kidney beans and turkey chili, accompanied by steamed broccoli.

Day 13:

Breakfast: A protein-rich smoothie consisting of spinach, bananas, almond milk, and protein powder.
Lunch consists of a whole-wheat tortilla wrapped around grilled veggies and hummus.
The supper consists of baked chicken breast, green beans, and roasted sweet potatoes.

Day 14:

Greek yogurt with peach slices and honey drizzled over it for breakfast.
Lunch consists of mixed greens with a lemon-tahini dressing, tuna, and white beans.
Quinoa tabbouleh and beef and vegetable kebabs for dinner.

Day 15:

Wholegrain oatmeal with sliced bananas and cinnamon on top for breakfast.
Lunch consists of a light Caesar dressing, romaine lettuce, and grilled chicken Caesar salad.
Supper is baked fish served over quinoa and roasted veggies.

Day 16:

Vegetarian frittata with bell peppers, onions, spinach, and feta cheese for breakfast.
Lunch consists of a mixed greens, cucumber, balsamic vinaigrette, and avocado and turkey salad.
Supper is brown rice, broccoli, and carrots stir-fried with tofu.

Day 17:

Smoothie bowl with granola, Greek yogurt, blended berries, and banana for breakfast.
Lunch consists of a mixed green salad and lentil soup served with whole-grain crackers on the side.
Dinner is wild rice, roasted Brussels sprouts, and grilled fish.

Day 18:

Whole-grain bread and scrambled eggs with sautéed mushrooms for breakfast.
Lunch consists of mixed greens, hummus, and a wrap with beans and veggies.
Roasted sweet potatoes and green beans paired with baked chicken thighs for dinner.

Day 19:

Greek yogurt parfait for breakfast, topped with chopped mango and shredded coconut.
Quinoa and black bean salad topped with cherry tomatoes, avocado, and lime vinaigrette for lunch.
Dinner consists of marinara-sauced turkey meatballs over zucchini noodles.

Day 20:

Waffles made with whole grains, topped with sliced strawberries and Greek yogurt for breakfast.
Lunch consists of mixed greens and quinoa salad alongside grilled shrimp skewers.
Brown rice, broccoli, and bell peppers stir-fried with beef for dinner.

Day 21:

Protein shake for breakfast, consisting of spinach, almond milk, banana, and protein powder.
Brown rice stir-fried with turkey and vegetables for lunch.
Supper consists of grilled chicken breast, quinoa, and roasted cauliflower.

Day 22:

Peach slices and a dash of cinnamon over cottage cheese for breakfast.
Lunch consists of mixed green salad on the side and lentil and vegetable soup.
Supper consists of baked cod fillet served with barley pilaf and steamed vegetables.

Day 23:

Wholegrain oatmeal with chopped walnuts and sliced bananas for breakfast.
Lunch: Chicken Caesar salad wrap with romaine lettuce, cherry tomatoes, and light Caesar dressing.
Brown rice, stir-fried veggies, and baked tofu for dinner.

Day 24:

Greek yogurt parfait with mixed berries and honey drizzled over it for breakfast.
Lunch consists of a salad of spinach and quinoa dressed with cucumber, grilled shrimp, and lemon-tahini sauce.
Steamed green beans on the side, along with turkey chili and kidney beans for dinner.

Day 25:

Vegetable scramble made with eggs, onions, bell peppers, and spinach for breakfast.
Lunch consists of a whole-wheat tortilla wrapped around grilled veggies and hummus.
Brown rice stir-fried with beef and broccoli for dinner.

Day 26:

Smoothie bowl with oats, Greek yogurt, blended mango, and pineapple for breakfast.
Lunch consists of a salad of avocado and chickpeas topped with cherry tomatoes, mixed greens, and balsamic vinaigrette.
Dinner is quinoa, roasted asparagus, and grilled fish.

Day 27:

Whole-grain bread and scrambled eggs with sautéed mushrooms for breakfast.
Lunch is lettuce wraps with tuna salad, cucumber, and avocado.
Dinner is wild rice, roasted Brussels sprouts, and baked chicken thighs.

Day 28:

Protein-rich smoothie for breakfast, made with protein powder, mixed berries, almond milk, and spinach.
Lunch consists of a mixed green salad and lentil soup served with whole-grain crackers on the side.
Steamed green beans and quinoa tabbouleh paired with grilled shrimp skewers for dinner.

Day 29:

Greek yogurt parfait for breakfast, topped with almonds, chopped apple, and honey drizzle.
Brown rice stir-fried with turkey and vegetables for lunch.
Supper consists of baked salmon served with quinoa and roasted cauliflower.

Day 30:

Protein smoothie bowl for breakfast with shredded coconut, chia seeds, and banana slices on top.
Lunch consists of mixed green salad, whole-grain bread, and lentil and vegetable soup.
Barley pilaf with grilled chicken breast and sautéed spinach for dinner.

Well done on finishing the 30-day meal plan! To effectively control your diabetes, don't forget to keep eating healthily and including regular exercise in your lifestyle. It's also critical to routinely check blood sugar levels and speak with a healthcare provider for individualized advice and assistance.

You've made great progress toward improving your diabetes management and fostering general health and well-being by adhering to this meal plan. To keep your meals interesting and fun, constantly experiment with different ingredients, flavors, and cooking techniques. Maintain your resolve, your erudition, and your commitment to your health path.

CHAPTER 10

MEASUREMENT AND CONVERSION CHART

A measurement and conversion table with common baking and culinary unit conversions:

1. Volume Measurements:

Five milliliters (ml) to one teaspoon (tsp)

15 milliliters (ml) / 1 tablespoon (tbsp)

30 milliliters (ml) are equal to one fluid ounce (fl oz).

A cup has 240 milliliters (ml) in it.

480 milliliters (ml) are equal to one pint (pt).

960 milliliters (ml) are equal to one quart (qt).

One gallon (gal) is equal to 3.8 liters (l).

2. Weight measurements:

1 pound (lb) = 16 ounces (oz) = 454 grams (g); 1 ounce (oz) = 28 grams (g)

1,000 grams (g) times one kilogram (kg) equals 2.2 pounds (lb).

3. Conversions of Temperature:

Celsius (°C) to Fahrenheit (°F): (°C × 9/5) + 32; - Fahrenheit (°F) to Celsius (°C): (°F - 32) × 5/9.

Water's freezing point is 32°F, or 0°C.
Water's boiling point is 212°F, or 100°C.

4. Common Kitchen Equivalents:

1/2 cup = 8 tablespoons = 4 ounces = 113 grams = 1 stick of butter

One medium egg is around 1/4 cup.

One medium onion is around one cup of chopped onion.

One clove of garlic, minced, equals around one teaspoon.

5. Oven Temperatures:

250°F to 325°F (120°C to 160°C) is the slow oven temperature.

Moderate oven: 160°C to 190°C, or 325°F to 375°F.

Hot oven: 190°C to 230°C (375°F to 450°F)

Extremely hot oven: 230°C (450°F) and higher

To guarantee precise quantities and conversions when baking and cooking, use this chart as a reference guide. It will assist you in more accurately following recipes and producing consistent outcomes while you cook.

INDEX

With the aid of this thorough index, readers will be able to quickly peruse your cookbook and locate the details and recipes they require to properly manage their diabetes and savor tasty, wholesome meals.

CONCLUSION

Let me conclude by sincerely congratulating you on starting this life-changing path to improved health and wellbeing. We've gone deeply into the complexities of managing diabetes throughout this cookbook, covering the subtleties of food selections, meal preparation, and lifestyle adjustments.

I hope that reading these pages has given you a sense of empowerment in addition to knowledge. Diabetes is a motivator for progress rather than an obstacle. You can take charge of your health and lead a full, energetic life by embracing a balanced diet, choosing foods carefully, and developing good eating habits.

Recall that your quest for wellbeing is only getting started with this cookbook. Every dish you make and every recipe you try is a chance to improve your physical and mental well-being and build resilience. You deserve to have a full and happy life since you are strong and capable.

May you always put your health first, pay attention to your body, and ask for help when you need it as you go. Remember that you are not on this path alone, and surround yourself with love, positivity, and encouragement. When we work together, we can conquer challenges, push past boundaries, and prosper in the face of hardship.

Winston Churchill once said, "It is the courage to persevere that counts. Failure is not fatal, and success is not final." Therefore, embrace your journey with bravery, tenacity, and unflinching confidence in your capacity to design the life you want.

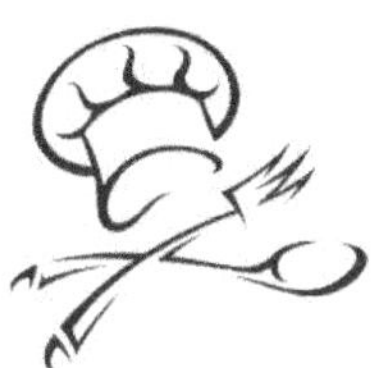
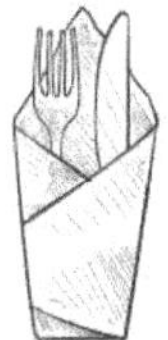

WEEKLY MEAL
PLANNER

WEEK:

DATE:

MONDAY

TUESDAY

SHOPPING LIST

WEDNESDAY

THURSDAY

FRIDAY

SATURDAY

SUNDAY

WEEKLY MEAL PLANNER

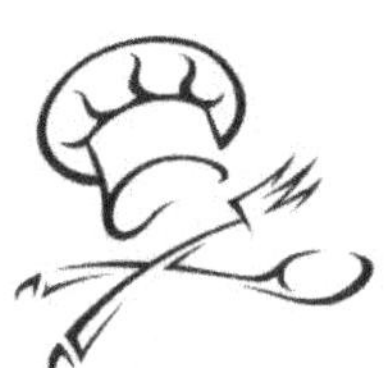

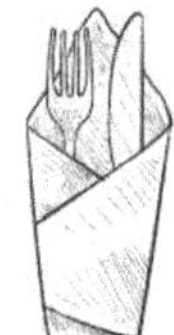

WEEK:

DATE:

MONDAY	TUESDAY	SHOPPING LIST
WEDNESDAY	THURSDAY	
FRIDAY	SATURDAY	

SUNDAY

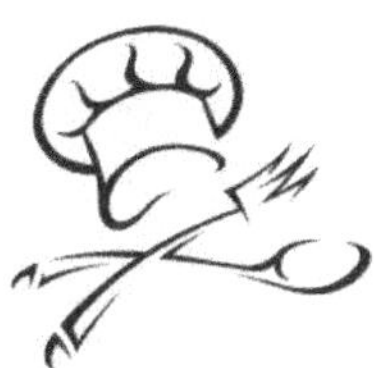

WEEKLY MEAL
PLANNER

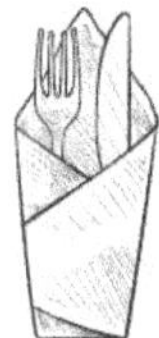

WEEK:

DATE:

MONDAY

TUESDAY

SHOPPING LIST

WEDNESDAY

THURSDAY

FRIDAY

SATURDAY

SUNDAY

WEEKLY MEAL
PLANNER

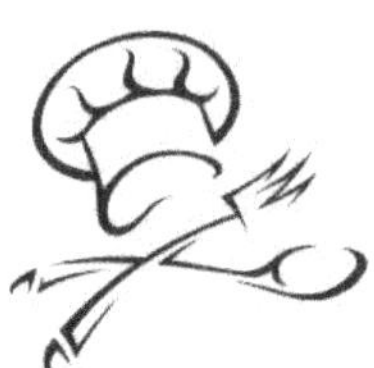
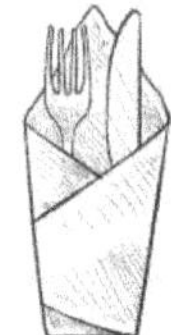

WEEK:

DATE:

MONDAY

TUESDAY

SHOPPING LIST

WEDNESDAY

THURSDAY

FRIDAY

SATURDAY

SUNDAY

WEEKLY MEAL
PLANNER

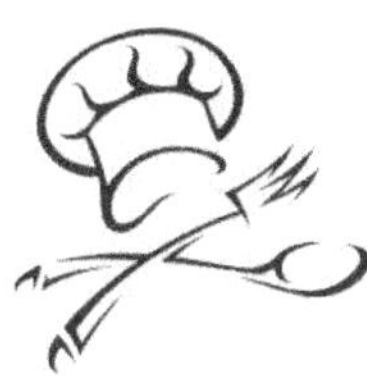
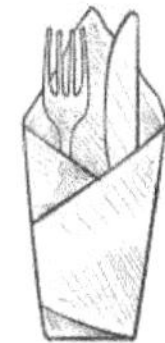

WEEK:

DATE:

MONDAY

TUESDAY

SHOPPING LIST

WEDNESDAY

THURSDAY

FRIDAY

SATURDAY

SUNDAY

WEEKLY MEAL PLANNER

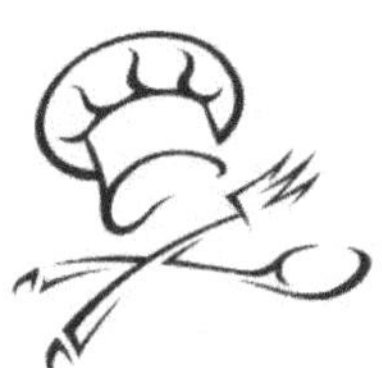

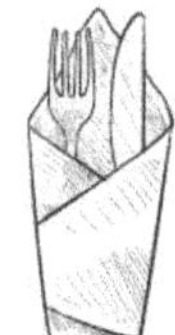

WEEK:

DATE:

MONDAY	TUESDAY	SHOPPING LIST

WEDNESDAY

THURSDAY

FRIDAY

SATURDAY

SUNDAY

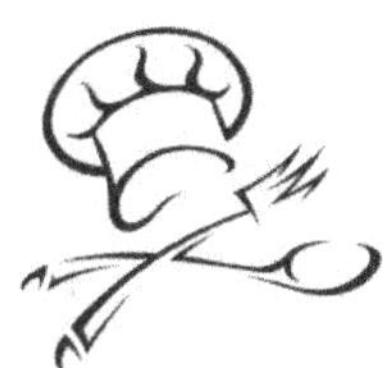

WEEKLY MEAL
PLANNER

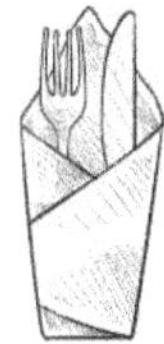

WEEK:

DATE:

MONDAY	TUESDAY	SHOPPING LIST
WEDNESDAY	THURSDAY	
FRIDAY	SATURDAY	
SUNDAY		

WEEKLY MEAL PLANNER

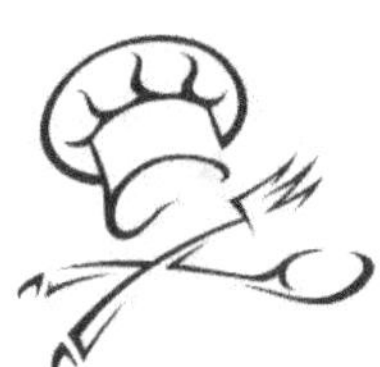

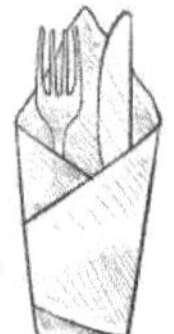

WEEK:

DATE:

MONDAY

TUESDAY

SHOPPING LIST

WEDNESDAY

THURSDAY

FRIDAY

SATURDAY

SUNDAY

WEEKLY MEAL
PLANNER

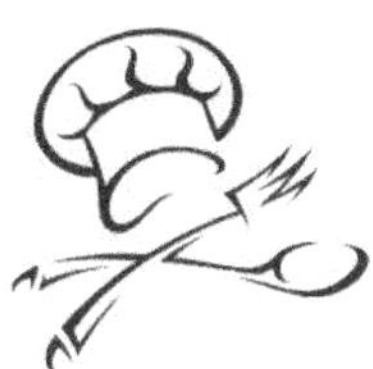
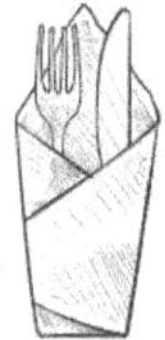

WEEK:

DATE:

MONDAY	TUESDAY

WEDNESDAY	THURSDAY

FRIDAY	SATURDAY

SUNDAY

SHOPPING LIST

WEEKLY MEAL PLANNER

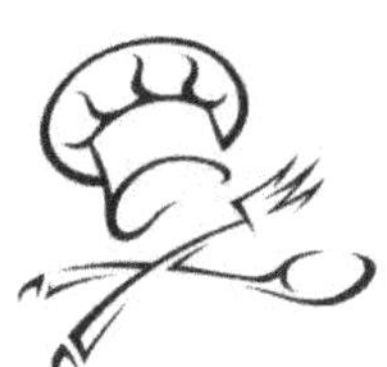
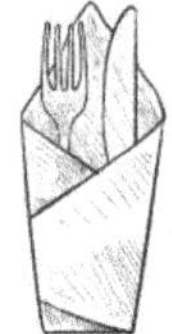

WEEK:

DATE:

MONDAY

TUESDAY

WEDNESDAY

THURSDAY

FRIDAY

SATURDAY

SUNDAY

SHOPPING LIST

WEEKLY MEAL PLANNER

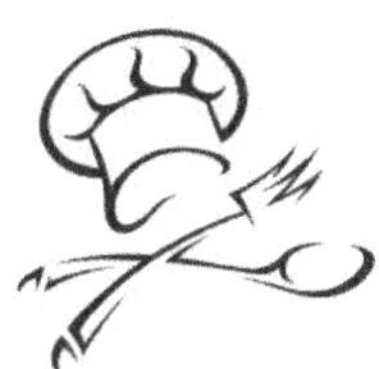

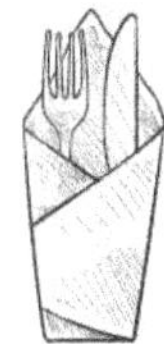

WEEK:

DATE:

MONDAY

TUESDAY

SHOPPING LIST

WEDNESDAY

THURSDAY

FRIDAY

SATURDAY

SUNDAY

WEEKLY MEAL PLANNER

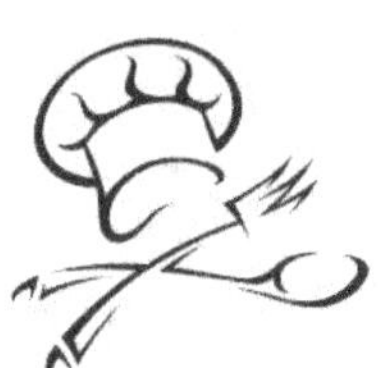
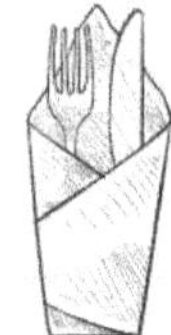

WEEK:

DATE:

MONDAY	TUESDAY	SHOPPING LIST
WEDNESDAY	THURSDAY	
FRIDAY	SATURDAY	

SUNDAY

WEEKLY MEAL
PLANNER

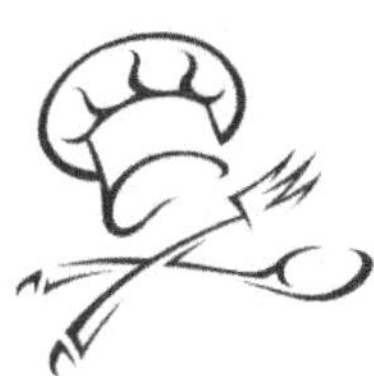
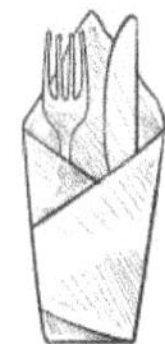

WEEK:

DATE:

MONDAY	TUESDAY	SHOPPING LIST
WEDNESDAY	THURSDAY	
FRIDAY	SATURDAY	
SUNDAY		

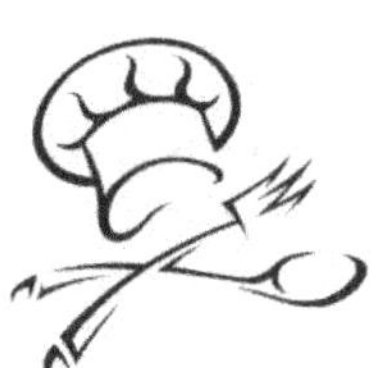

WEEKLY MEAL
PLANNER

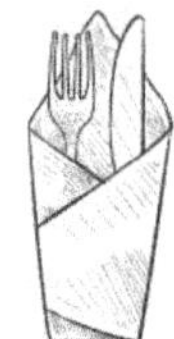

WEEK:

DATE:

MONDAY

TUESDAY

SHOPPING LIST

WEDNESDAY

THURSDAY

FRIDAY

SATURDAY

SUNDAY

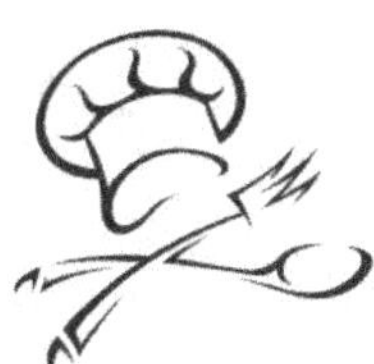

WEEKLY MEAL
PLANNER

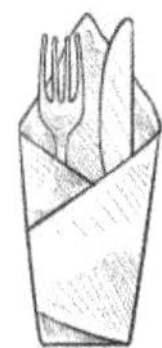

WEEK:

DATE:

MONDAY	TUESDAY	SHOPPING LIST

WEDNESDAY	THURSDAY	

FRIDAY	SATURDAY	

SUNDAY

WEEKLY MEAL
PLANNER

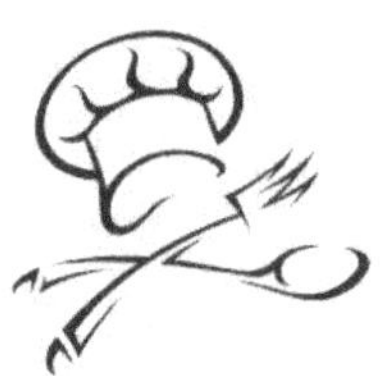
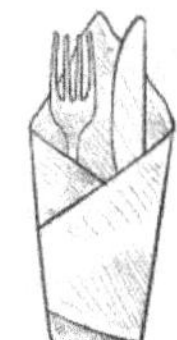

WEEK:

DATE:

MONDAY	TUESDAY	SHOPPING LIST

WEDNESDAY	THURSDAY

FRIDAY	SATURDAY

SUNDAY

WEEKLY MEAL
PLANNER

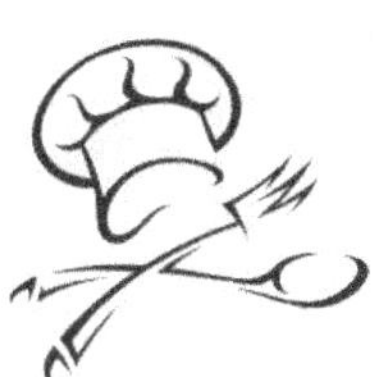
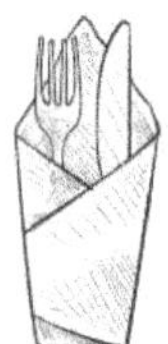

WEEK:

DATE:

MONDAY	TUESDAY	SHOPPING LIST

WEDNESDAY	THURSDAY

FRIDAY	SATURDAY

SUNDAY

WEEKLY MEAL
PLANNER

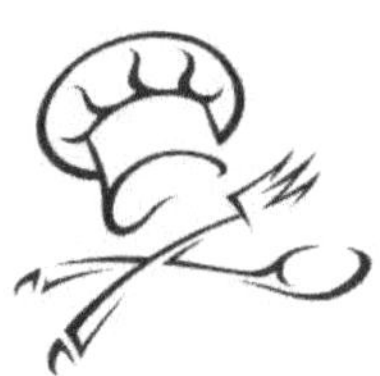
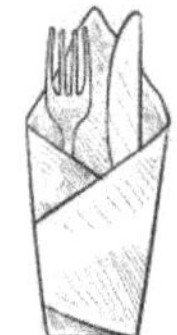

WEEK:

DATE:

MONDAY

TUESDAY

SHOPPING LIST

WEDNESDAY

THURSDAY

FRIDAY

SATURDAY

SUNDAY

WEEKLY MEAL PLANNER

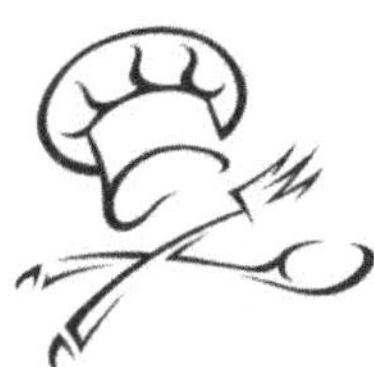

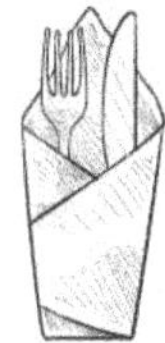

WEEK:

DATE:

MONDAY

TUESDAY

WEDNESDAY

THURSDAY

FRIDAY

SATURDAY

SUNDAY

SHOPPING LIST

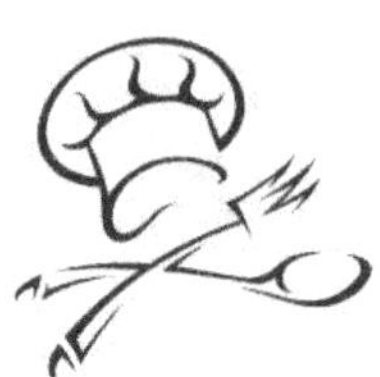

WEEKLY MEAL
PLANNER

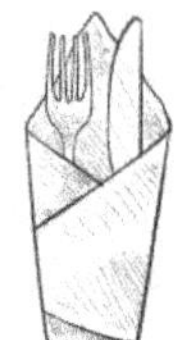

WEEK:

DATE:

MONDAY

TUESDAY

SHOPPING LIST

WEDNESDAY

THURSDAY

FRIDAY

SATURDAY

SUNDAY

WEEKLY MEAL
PLANNER

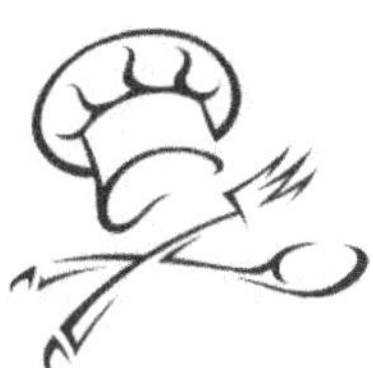

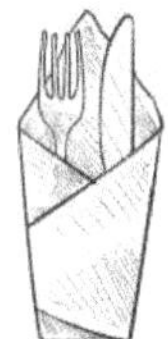

WEEK:

DATE:

MONDAY

TUESDAY

SHOPPING LIST

WEDNESDAY

THURSDAY

FRIDAY

SATURDAY

SUNDAY